The Myth of Primary Polydipsia:

Why Hypovolemic Dehydration Can Explain the Real Physiological Basis of So-Called 'Psychogenic Water Drinking'

Patrick Ussher

This book is dedicated to all those patients who are currently suffering from a continuous and, at times, life-threatening nightmare of perpetual thirst in the hope that their suffering can at last cease.

And, again, this book is dedicated to the memory of my mum, Mary Redmond-Ussher (1950-2015) whose Pink Ribbon Path *inspires me every day.*

About the Author

Patrick Ussher is a composer of music in a contemporary classical style. His music is part of the *Artlist* catalogue and can also be listened to on Spotify. He is also the author of *Stoicism & Western Buddhism: A Reflection on Two Philosophical Ways of Life* and *POTS: What It Really Is & Why It Happens*. A founding member of the Modern Stoicism project, an interdisciplinary collaboration between academics and psychothera-pists working to create modern applications of the ancient Greco-Roman philosophy of Stoicism, he started and ran the project's blog from 2012 to 2016. As part of the Modern Stoicism project, he also edited two books: *Stoicism Today: Selected Writings, Volumes 1 & 2.* In 2018, he worked with Columba Press on a new edition of a book by his late mother, Mary Redmond-Ussher, on coping with breast cancer under the title *Following the Pink Ribbon Path*. Patrick has a BA and MA in Classics (Ancient Greek & Latin) from the University of Exeter, UK. He has also recently written a pseudonymous political satire. His website is: www.patrickussher.com

'The diagnosis of compulsive water drinking must be made with care and may represent our ignorance of yet undescribed pathophysiological mechanisms.'

'The understanding of the pathophysiology of this disease has made little progress [since Barlow and De Wardener's paper].'

- Prof. Daniel Bichet in Melmed S., Ed. *The Pituitary (4th Edition)*, 2017.

'It is customary and reasonable to consider that compulsive water drinking occurs in emotionally disturbed people.'

- Barlow & De Wardener, 'Compulsive Water Drinking', *Quarterly Journal of Medicine*, 1959.

Table of Contents

Introduction

A t this very moment, there are many people worldwide who are stuck in a cycle of excessive thirst and urination. Their symptoms constitute a kind of perpetual hell: their bodies scream with thirst but, no matter how much they drink, that thirst cannot be quenched. They drink in large quantities of water and urinate out large quantities of dilute urine. Some drink so much water that their blood sodium levels become dangerously low to the point of developing hyponatraemia. Of these, a minority may even go into a hyponatraemia-induced coma in which their brain swells from the excessive water in their system. And, of these, some will die.

When these patients present to the hospital, they will likely be placed in acute care. The medics will scramble to try and work out why these patients are suffering from excessive thirst. Do they have Type II Diabetes? No, their blood sugars are normal. What about kidney damage? No, all kidney markers are normal. Could they have Diabetes Insipidus, a rare condition in which the brain cannot produce much or any of the water retention hormone, vasopressin (also known as 'anti-diuretic hormone')? No, the water deprivation test has resulted in concentrated urine: this means their body was always capable of conserving water and that, therefore, their vasopressin release is intact. This means that the only other possible diagnosis is....'Primary Polydipsia'.

Primary Polydipsia is currently considered to be a psychiatric condition in which patients drink excessive quantities of fluids for no possible physiological reason (indeed, the word 'Primary', in this instance, means that there is no physiological cause). If vasopressin can work, or so the thinking goes, then there can exist no reason to drink so much water: after all, the body was always capable of conserving it. The very same patients I described above are, under this view therefore, stuck in a hell purely of their own making. Most likely these patients are mentally ill and their emotionally disturbed state somehow 'manifests' in a compulsion to drink excessive fluids. Sadly, medics will say to each other, it is very hard to help these patients. Even after their hyponatraemia is corrected, they will usually return to their compulsive water drinking. What can be done with such people?

In this book, I will argue that the underlying premise behind Primary Polydipsia is profoundly flawed and that the condition, as it is currently understood, is the result of a catastrophic error rooted in long outdated ideas that owe far more to Freud than to science. Furthermore, I will suggest that the patients I have described above are not drinking large quantities of water because they are mentally ill but because of a serious and devastating pathophysiology. And that some of these patients are dying not because of an inexplicable compulsion to drink too much water but because they are suffering from an organic state of physical ill-health that carries a significant risk of fatality.

This book necessarily focusses on the harms that medics can cause when they view their patients' suffering as psychological. Freud's long and cruel shadow has much to answer for and, despite the unscientific nature of many of his ideas, his legacy still informs much of modern medical practice when it encounters symptoms that it does not yet understand. It is hubristic to believe that everything about the human body has already been understood. The effort to understand health and disease will go on for as long as humanity survives. Symptoms that are as yet mysterious should be viewed as clarion calls to return to the drawing board. To throw your hands up in the air and claim such symptoms are psychosomatic is to take the easy way out.

However, while the harms that are currently being done to so-called Primary Polydiptics are undeniable and, objectively-speaking, amount to medical negligence, they are not the product of malevolence but of a limited understanding of what these patients are really facing. Doctors generally go into their profession in order to heal and save lives but, sometimes, this aspiration will be blocked by inadequate knowledge. In this case, that 'block' stems from the strong psychiatric influence that shaped the initial thinking about Primary Polydipsia. Indeed, the first medics who observed so-called 'compulsive water drinkers' believed strongly in 'conversion disorders' or in the capacity of female hysteria to cause just about any symptom under the sun. These ideas were part of the zeitgeist of the time. On the other hand, far fewer physicians would believe in them today. The very fact that Primary Polydipsia was first conceptualised through such a psychiatric lens should be enough to lead any medical researcher to be curious about whether its current premises are well-founded or whether, perhaps, something else might be going on.

Furthermore, psychosomatic understandings of poorly understood symptoms rarely age well. Multiple Sclerosis and Parkinson's were once viewed in such a light before the degradation of myelin, the protective sheath around the brain, and the lowered output of dopamine, were discovered as having their respective causal roles. Similarly, ME/CFS (Myalgic Encephalomyelitis / Chronic Fatigue Syndrome) patients have faced the same stigma. Over decades, however, and in particular more recently, research is unravelling the complex pathophysiology that underlies this illness also. Indeed, the research into ME/CFS will form a central part of this book as it is this illness, I believe, which holds the clue to demystifying Primary Polydipsia. This is because a significant number of ME/CFS patients suffer from extreme thirst and, just like in so-called Primary Polydipsia, produce large quantities of dilute urine with a tendency towards hyponatraemia. Is there a kind of polydipsia which is largely specific to ME/CFS (and closely related illnesses), the precise mechanisms of which are yet to be mapped out, and which may in fact be what has always been mistakenly termed 'psychogenic water drinking'? The answer to this question is particularly important as most of the mechanisms identified in Long Covid have also been found in ME/CFS, a fact that leads many researchers to regard them as the same illness. If I am right, therefore, to suggest that the answer to Primary Polydipsia is to be found in ME/CFS, then the problem of clarifying the exact nature of the extreme thirst under discussion becomes even more urgent as it is likely that the number of people suffering from this symptom will have risen exponentially since the recent pandemic (indeed, as we shall see in chapter two when we discuss the similarities between ME/CFS and Long Covid, extreme thirst is a commonly reported symptom by Long Covid patients).

But why am I writing this book?

At one level, I am writing this book both because I feel for the suffering of those who are still stuck in the continuous nightmare of this symptom and because I believe strongly that it is possible to reverse it. At the moment, no substantive help is offered to these patients. In this book, I aim to present a compelling argument for a new form of polydipsia which, if validated, could pave the way for successful treatments and the mitigation of suffering.

At another level, this book is aimed at counteracting the stigma that is currently attached to Primary Polydipsia. It is bad enough that patients should receive no real guidance as to how to relieve their symptoms but that they should also be blamed as the sole cause of their suffering is cruel in the extreme, particularly when one considers that such patients are likely to be held responsible even for their own deaths. The 'blame the victim' nature of the diagnosis might also lead to a reduction in support from the family and friends of the patient in question, an unfortunate by-product of a culture which values the opinion of 'the experts' at all costs, even in situations where that expert opinion is highly illogical and ill-founded (as I believe applies in this case). As a result, the very ill may receive less familial support and become ever more isolated.

But that I should come to write this book in the first place is because of a highly personal reason. Indeed, when I mentioned, just above, that I empathised with those who were 'still stuck in the nightmare of this continuous symptom', it is because I too was once stuck in that nightmare. And I will now describe exactly what that nightmare is like.

The Story of a 'Primary Polydipsia' Patient

I was diagnosed with Primary Polydipsia.

I know what it is like to go through symptoms from hell as a result of which I often felt I would not see the morning light. To feel that there was no escape from the terrifying reality in which I was trapped and that there was no way my body could take much more of the strain it was under. That it was unlikely I would make it to my 32nd birthday.

And I know what it is like to be hospitalised with these very symptoms and then to be viewed as having them because I was supposedly 'mentally ill'. To try to describe what I was going through but not to be taken seriously. To hear a doctor and a nurse laughing about their Primary Polydipsia case in the hallway. And afterwards to talk to family members about the 'diagnosis' only to be met with awkward silences or statements to the effect that the experts must be right and, anyway, they saved your life, so really you should just be grateful.

The fact is that, because of the belief that Primary Polydipsia is caused by mental illness, physicians tend to disregard what their patients try to communicate about their symptoms. After all, how can such people be trusted to convey accurately what they sense in their bodies?

But there is one thing that so-called Primary Polydiptics will say the world over, namely that they are *thirsty*. Not just a little thirsty but extremely thirsty. Dying of thirst, in fact (and this is not merely a metaphor). To those who believe that Primary Polydipsia is caused by mental illness, I ask you this: how mentally ill does someone have to be to misread such a basic bodily signal so profoundly? And is it really that likely that the countless numbers of such patients worldwide who complain of this extreme thirst are all *that* mentally ill?

I can tell you quite clearly that the thirst is real. My body screamed with thirst. Every muscle ached with thirst. On the worst nights, the ones where I thought I was going to die, my muscles would twitch and spasm, I felt that blood was not reaching my brain, that I was fading away, that this was it. And always, always the terrible thirst. I could urinate 10 litres on such nights. Once I did not sleep for three nights out of four. All I could do during those times was try to keep the smile of my late mother in my mind and hope to make it to the morning. But the image was faint, very, very faint. And my body felt like it wanted to let go of life.

Except it didn't. It hung on. And once the morning light came, all I could do was stay in bed, keep very still and hope that I would be granted at least some sleep the next night. It would take several days of lying still like this to become somewhat more stable and for the thirst to lessen to a more manageable level.

But these extreme episodes would come back, never randomly but, crucially as I shall explain later in this introduction, always triggered by physical over-exertion (the classic symptom exacerbator in ME/CFS, an illness I had developed a few years previously). I must have had a dozen such episodes over six months before, on the last such occasion, I decided I had to get to a hospital. As I left the door of my apartment, I had no idea if I would return. I knew I couldn't manage the situation myself anymore and, indeed, I feared that I was going to die if I didn't receive medical attention: I needed to be in a hospital bed. I also knew, with a heavy heart, that I would probably end up being diagnosed with Primary Polydipsia – after all, as I had read in online patient forums, excessively thirsty patients with my chronic illness tend to be told that that is what their problem really is. But I also knew that it was a risk I had to take if I was to survive and, I told myself, there was always a chance that I might have Diabetes Insipidus, a condition that needs life-long treatment.

In the process of triage at A&E, it was found that my blood sodium level was 116. The normal range is 135-144. At that level of blood sodium, I could easily have been in a coma or dead. The first doctor to examine me suggested that I most likely had Primary Polydipsia. He explained to me that if I had Diabetes Insipidus, I would be by hyper- rather than hyponatraemic (this is because where the body cannot produce any vasopressin at all, the patient loses all available free water, leading to internal dehydration). Interestingly, he also said that Primary Polydiptics are often helped by drinking electrolyte drinks. Why this should be the case fits well with the overall thesis of this book, as we shall see, but it doesn't make much sense if it is true that so-called Primary Polydipsia patients are drinking excessive fluids for psychological reasons. Such patients should, after all, knock back any old drink, whatever it might be.

The next day, things suddenly took a turn for the worse, however. My blood sodium levels auto-corrected too quickly and, fearing the risk of cerebral damage (which is a known complication of overly rapid correction of blood sodium), it was decided that my bloodstream needed to be diluted again by the use of an IV drip and Desmopressin injections. The following week was extremely challenging. Blood tests were taken every two hours, morning and night (I doubt I got more than eight hours sleep in total that whole week). Eventually, it was decided that the risk of cerebral swelling had ended and that I was to start the water deprivation test, the most common test used to distinguish between whether someone has Primary Polydipsia or Diabetes Insipidus. If someone can't concentrate their urine, vasopressin release is so impaired that

Diabetes Insipidus is diagnosed. If they can concentrate their urine then, or so the thinking goes, there was never any physiological need to have been drinking so much water in the first place (as their body was always capable of conserving it).

As someone who was accustomed to drinking between 6-8 litres of water on my good days, and up to 20 litres over 24 hours on a bad day, the idea of drinking nothing at all for an extended period seemed utterly terrifying. Indeed, frankly, it seemed crazy. But the experience, as difficult as it was to tolerate, was to change my life forever and for the better, albeit not for the reasons my doctors might have expected.

I stopped drinking at 10 PM the night before the test. By midday of the next day, my body was really struggling. My heartrate was over 120 lying in bed and I felt very ill and faint. But I did my best to cope with the situation. And at 4 PM something unexpected happened: I suddenly felt less thirsty. The thirst was still there but it was no longer raging, no longer all encompassing. At the exact same time, my blood sodium levels returned to the normal range and my urine began to concentrate. I had not seen anything but dilute urine in a very long time. Although the significance of this moment escaped me at the time, the fact that normally concentrated blood lessened my thirst strikes me as a major clue as to what is likely really going on in this condition (as we will explore further later on and, in particular, in chapter four).

From my perspective, I was utterly overjoyed at this change. I communicated this to the team. I relished only sipping water. I was so happy no longer to be so thirsty, it felt like a miracle. For the rest of my time in hospital, I drank only a glass here or there and probably less than anyone else in my ward.

At the very same moment however that I ceased drinking large amounts of water and communicated my relief that I was no longer so thirsty, the team concluded that the result meant that I definitely had Primary Polydipsia. After all, the water deprivation test had 'proved' this diagnosis (in that my urine could become concentrated due to the release of vasopressin) and this is clearly more important than the behaviour of the patient. In some ways, I think that this moment epitomizes the ludicrousness of the thinking that currently underpins Primary Polydipsia: what the textbook has to say matters more than what the patient reports and their behaviour.

As I mentioned above, I knew that I was being treated as a mental case throughout my stay in the hospital. In retrospect, I wish I had spoken up for myself more and pointed out the obvious inconsistences between my experience and the way I was being viewed. At various different times, I was told 'You are only in here because you were drinking too much water' or 'Don't drink water behind our back when you go to the toilet'. And, of course, overhearing the doctor and nurse in the hall laughing about the fact that I supposedly had Primary Polydipsia.

I had mentioned a research paper into ME/CFS which demonstrated that water and salt retaining hormones tended to be downregulated in the illness. I had no real conception, at that point, as to why excessive thirst occurred in my illness but perhaps this paper was somehow relevant to my situation? But the doctors in the hospital knew nothing about ME/CFS and they would also have been admittedly hard-pressed, in a busy hospital environment, to reflect on how ME/CFS might have been driving my symptoms. Later on, though, I learnt that they had never really taken my points about ME/CFS seriously. My medical records, which I requested a couple of years later, stated that I felt I had ME/CFS due to 'non-specific symptoms' (although I had tried to explain both post-exertional malaise and hypovolemia) and that I was 'admitted with self-diagnosed ME' (something which is untrue, I had been diagnosed several years prior although it was later doubly confirmed by a specialist). The fact is that, given that my early symptom presentation accorded with that which is seen in so-called Primary Polydipsia, my fate was clearly sealed from the beginning.

But I was doing better and so I put these things aside. I was out of hospital and, despite the general situation that I have just described, I was still very grateful to the medical team who had likely saved my life. As I also read in my medical records some years later, there had been a point at which moving me to intensive care was on the cards. As much as I believe that my real problem went unrecognised in that hospital, they did their best, according to the protocols and procedures they had been taught, to get me out of the life-threatening situation that I was in. I had gone into hospital with a blood sodium level of 116 and I left it with that level restored to the normal range. Although the diagnosis was humiliating and I felt myself to be largely unheard throughout my time in hospital, I remain grateful for the central aspects of the care I received, a care which ultimately set me on a path to a better quality of life. I still had ME/CFS but the worst of my thirst seemed to be over.

But it was not gone completely. It remained, light but discernible. However, I did my best to ignore it. I was so thrilled to be able to drink a more normal amount of water that the slight thirst didn't bother me. Two weeks after leaving the hospital, however, I physically overextended and experienced an episode of post-exertional malaise. At exactly the same time, the thirst came roaring back (not as extreme as previously, nothing could be, but still the thirst was strong and unquenchable). It was particularly bad at night. I tried drinking more water at such times but this risked, it soon became clear, the same old vicious cycle. I carefully limited my fluid intake, keen to avoid going down the previous path. 'Why is this happening?', I wondered to myself. 'Maybe I am just a crazy Primary Polydipsia patient after all'.

But this hypothesis, which I seriously considered, did not make sense. Why did the thirst become so strong while in an episode of post-exertional malaise? And why was it manageable at other times? Something physiological had to be going on and it must have been something to do with my illness. For those unfamiliar with ME/CFS (and I will delve in more detail into its pathophysiology in chapter two), post-exertional malaise (or PEM) is its central symptom. A whole range of abnormalities make exercise difficult for those with the illness and overextending beyond one's physical capacities results in often severe symptoms. Depending on how badly affected the patient is by the illness, they may then spend hours, days or weeks largely in bed or housebound. I have experienced such episodes well over a hundred times. The symptoms involved can be very unpleasant and debilitating. And, as if on cue, the thirst will arrive: strong and unquenchable.

I was feeling at a loss but I knew I had to work something out. I didn't want the nightmare to start up again. Why are some ME/CFS patients so thirsty? This was the question I had to answer. And I knew I was not the only one. I will describe what experts in the field have to say about this symptom in chapter three, as well as patient testimonies, but for now it is relevant to mention that I had read hundreds of accounts of patients in online forums complaining of extreme thirst, some drinking 6, 8, 10 or (many) more litres per day. And their thirst sounded just like mine: unquenchable with a tendency towards dilute urine and hyponatraemia. Something else had to be going on.

After my experience in the hospital, I had wanted to learn more about hyponatraemia and so I had purchased a book by Prof. Tim Noakes entitled *Waterlogged*. The book focussed on the dangers of overhydration during sport. The advice for athletes to keep their fluids up while engaging in long-distance runs, for example, can be dangerous as, during strenuous physical activity, the kidneys cannot excrete water effectively. This can lead to a build-up of free water in the system and result in hyponatraemia. There have been many tragic cases of athletes who drop into a coma and even die as a result of the misplaced advice to 'keep the fluids up' during exercise. Prof. Noakes is one pioneer in the general effort to educate the athletic public about such dangers.

Early on in the book, there was a diagram giving an overview of thirst physiology. The bulk of it was focussed on explaining how osmotic thirst works. This is the only kind of thirst most healthy people will ever experience. Their urine becomes darker, they don't have enough free water in the system, and the osmotic thirst centre generates a thirst signal. The solution is simply to drink more water.

But it was on this diagram that I spotted something else, something I had never heard of (although I had sometimes wondered if it existed): the hypovolemic thirst centre. This thirst centre has a very different role and it is triggered when blood volume drops by 10%. This is the thirst signal the body creates when it does not have enough blood.

My mind raced furiously and made all kinds of connections. What had been completely baffling and mysterious was suddenly rendered, at least potentially, comprehensible. What if I had suffered extreme thirst not because I was short on water but because I did not have enough blood?

This might strike the reader as an odd question to ponder. After all, how can a human being, when not suffering from an open and gushing wound or some kind of major fluid loss from vomiting for example, possibly not have enough blood?

But I knew, from reading the research, that ME/CFS patients often do indeed not have enough blood. In fact, the research has clearly shown that low blood volume, as we shall explore in chapter two, is a key characteristic of the illness, with a subset of patients typically at least one litre short of blood (in other words, they usually have around four litres of blood while a healthy person has around five). This largely, though not entirely, occurs because there is a downregulation of the usual hormonal mechanisms by which the body can boost and maintain blood levels. Even more relevant to my situation was that I knew that those very same mechanisms tended to become even further downregulated during episodes of post-exertional malaise, leading to increased salt loss and even lower blood volume during those times, a factor that could potentially explain why I experienced my worst thirst during such episodes.

My eyes then latched onto something else in Noakes' book. Next to the hypovolemic thirst centre were the words 'salt + water appetite'. This means that the hypovolemic thirst centre cannot be quenched by the drinking of water alone: in order to increase blood volume, the body needs appropriately concentrated fluids. Blood is concentrated stuff, after all.

Things suddenly became clearer and clearer: what had I been doing but drinking copious amounts of water in response to the thirst I felt? What if my thirst was indeed driven by an organic pathology but I had been unwittingly applying the wrong solution to the problem? The water I drank could never boost blood volume: it is the prerogative of the kidneys to filter water out of the system in a timely manner. A new model emerged in my mind for why I had experienced my symptoms:

> Hypovolemic state >>> Hypovolemic thirst centre activates >>> drink water >>> water urinated out >>> low blood volume remains along with related thirst >>> repeat vicious cycle.

In light of this model, I then developed an alternative hypothesis for treating my symptoms:

> Hypovolemic state >>> hypovolemic thirst centre activates >>> drink appropriately concentrated fluids >>> blood volume is boosted and hypovolemic thirst centre is quenched >>> repeat so as to keep hypovolemic thirst at bay.

I needed to test this hypothesis as soon as possible but how could I do so? I remembered a recent study by Medow et al. (which we will consider in more detail in chapter four) in which the effect of drinking ORS (Oral Rehydration Solution) on boosting blood volume was studied. These are packets of glucose mixed with salt and potassium, most typically taken during episodes of diarrhoea in order to counteract the fluid loss that accompanies such episodes. The sachets have other uses too though. Indeed, the presence of glucose in the solution acts to transport nearly all of the salt across the gut and directly into the bloodstream, where it then stays temporarily, thereby effectively boosting blood volume. We will consider exactly how this mechanism works in chapter four but, in essence, ORS is somewhat akin to having a saline IV in your pocket. I immediately went out to the nearby pharmacy, bought a box of Dioralyte, and drank 600 ml of the stuff.

The thirst went away. Not only did the thirst go away but the lights switched back on. I could get up the stairs more easily as my heart had more blood to work with. My nervous system also calmed down noticeably (I later learnt that low blood volume is a very stressful state of affairs for the brain).

Eureka! I had worked it out. I now understood that my thirst had really been caused by not having enough blood, a central component of my chronic illness. I also understood, at last, why my thirst had got worse while in episodes of post-exertional malaise as, at those times, my body experienced additional solute loss. And, most importantly of all, Primary Polydipsia clearly did not apply to me: I had just been applying the wrong solution to my real, physiological problem. Indeed, maybe, I wondered to myself, Primary Polydipsia itself was based on misguided ideas. Was it really a well-validated condition with plenty of convincing research behind it? What was the history of this, on the face of it, rather odd idea that people, who claimed to be dying of thirst, were actually stuck in some strange psychological compulsion to spend every waking hour downing enormous quantities of water?

But I left those thoughts alone for a long time. The whole experience had been deeply traumatic – indeed, I developed PTSD as a result of my extreme symptoms, something which still affects me today. I was just

14

glad to find a way to manage the thirst at long last and wanted to put the whole experience behind me. I was so delighted only to need around 2.5 litres of fluid per day and to find a simple medical solution that had a quasi-miraculous effect on the thirst I experienced (I will describe further the kinds of self-devised protocols I ended up following to manage my hypovolemic dehydration in more detail in chapter four). I still had ME/CFS but the biggest nightmare associated with it was, at last, over.

But a couple of years later, a voice was still nagging away at me: what if 'Primary Polydipsia' is a mistake? What if it has always been hypovolemic dehydration by another name? I was also aware that, if my ideas about hypovolemic dehydration were correct, many very ill people were suffering needlessly and were also being erroneously stigmatised by the doctors to whom they turned for help.

So I plucked up my courage and began to research the literature, both historical and current, about Primary Polydipsia. As a result, I was soon struck (or perhaps 'shocked' is a better word) by three things in particular.

Firstly, the condition is clearly the product of the very worst kinds of 'psychosomatising-psychiatry'. Indeed, those who first formulated the condition attributed variously its causes to such staples as: conversion disorders, hysterical fugues, delusional hypochondriasis, female hysteria, not having enough sex, troubled marriages and so on. The early literature concerning Primary Polydipsia is, in fact, a parody of itself. I very much doubt that most current medics are aware of the condition's history. Rather, when discussed in medical school, I would imagine that it is taught in purely practical terms: the utility of the water deprivation test, the significance of dilute urine in the context of hypo- rather than of hypernatremia and so on. If modern-day medics were aware of the condition's history, I imagine that most would think twice about its supposed assumptions.

The second striking thing is how little interest the condition has received. A lifetime PubMed search for "Psychogenic Polydipsia" yields only 284 results while, by way of contrast, a search for "Multiple Sclerosis" returns 101,484 results. This lack of interest, extraordinary when one considers that so-called Primary Polydipsia can result in serious complications and even in death, also does not speak to a condition that is on strong theoretical grounds. It is not an illness that has had the necessary conditions for advances in scientific understanding, namely rigorous debate and criticism. Rather, its early assumptions quickly became ossified and nearly all subsequent research, operating from within those same assumptions, has done nothing other than the equivalent of a team of explorers who, stubbornly clearing the same path in a jungle for months on end, wonder why it is that they are still lost.

The third striking thing is that 'Primary Polydipsia' was conceptualised in a time of limited medical knowledge. By this, I refer specifically to the fact that the hypovolemic thirst centre was not discovered, as we shall see in chapter two, until the 1960s, long after the idea of 'psychogenic water drinking' had taken hold. This means that the early researchers of so-called Primary Polydipsia were hampered by not having enough physiological knowledge. I believe that the concept of hypovolemic dehydration can explain entirely a polydipsia with a tendency towards dilute urine and hyponatraemia: the results of applying the wrong solution to the problem. However, if you take the hypovolemic thirst centre out of the picture and you are only aware of the osmotic thirst centre, then the behaviour of so-called Primary Polydipsia patients will, indeed, appear to be mentally ill.

Considering all of these factors, I came to be strongly of the view that Primary Polydipsia was formulated at a time when no one could possibly have known the real reasons for the thirst which these patients experienced and, as a result, it was simply assumed that the problem must be psychological: the same old, hubristic medical error that so many patients have had to suffer in other contexts. The lens through which the condition was conceived was, therefore, wrong. As a result, its diagnostic procedures and treatments were also wrong. The current formulations around the condition represent a classic case of getting the wrong answers because of asking the wrong questions.

And that is why I am writing this book, so as to look at so-called Primary Polydipsia from an entirely new angle, one which takes the finding of the hypovolemic thirst centre into account and which keeps Freud, and his kind, firmly out of the picture. This whole book is an attempt to answer the question: 'If these patients were to be examined for the very first time today, knowing what we know now, how could we explain their symptoms?'

I should make clear, however, that this book is not challenging some aspects of the current thinking on Primary Polydipsia. The first aspect is that there are, despite everything I have just said, some people who do indeed drink excessive amounts of water for purely psychological reasons. In other words, some people drink a large amount of water because they 'think' they need to do so. Typically, such patients might regard it as important to drink a lot of water for health reasons although their reasons can be more specific. For example, one elderly man was told to drink 'plenty of water' as part of his recovery from an urological surgery. The result was that, taking the advice very literally, he drank 8 litres of water in 24 hours and developed a hyponatraemic seizure.[1] In another case, a middle-aged woman experienced withdrawal symptoms from stopping benzodiazepine and, on the advice of a neighbour, started to increase her water intake. She then developed cerebral edema.[2] A third example is the case of a man who drank up to 3 gallons of water

1. Han et al., 'Hyponatraemic seizure secondary to primary polydipsia following urological surgery', 2022.

2. Utzon et al., 'Psychogenic polydipsia: pronounced cerebral edema after exaggerated consumption of boiled water', 1991.

daily purely in order to suppress his chronic hiccups. He developed a blood sodium level of 111 and required hospitalisation.[3] A final example comes from back in 1959 when a 16 year old man was admitted to Beth Israel hospital in New York. He had upped his food intake so as to bulk up and impress his older girlfriend. His medical team noted, however, that after a period 'he felt that his weight gain had been excessive and, in order to decrease food consumption, he voluntarily began to ingest large quantities of fluid. He did not complain of excessive thirst, and had no particular preference for iced liquids.'[4]

When we consider these examples, it is clear that, in one sense, Primary Polydipsia as it is currently understood, does exist: psychogenic water drinking can be a thing. However, the key characteristic of such patients is that they do *not* suffer from excessive thirst: they have their reasons for drinking so much water but biological thirst is not one of them. Therefore, this true 'psychogenic water drinking' is entirely separate from my concern in this book, namely patients who complain of a raging and all-encompassing thirst and whose suffering is nevertheless currently psychologised. Indeed, given that 'polydipsia' is a term that implies excessive thirst, one wonders if true psychogenic water drinking should be classified as a kind of polydipsia at all, given the absence of reported thirst, and whether it should perhaps be termed something else altogether, maybe using a term that just implies that it is a misguided behaviour or habit.

The second aspect of current thinking on Primary Polydipsia that this book does not, at least intentionally, set out to challenge refers to a specific subset of Primary Polydipsia that has been identified in patients with schizophrenia. This subset is separated out by experts from the

---

3. Ramirez and Graham, 'Hiccups, Compulsive Water Drinking, and Hyponatremia', 1993.

4. Wedeen, 'Prolonged functional depression of antidiuretic mechanisms in psychogenic polydipsia simulating primary diabetes insipidus', 1961.

more typical 'psychogenic water drinking' and, while the reasons for increased fluid consumption in schizophrenics remain unknown, it does seem to be the case that schizophrenics can suffer from specific patho-physiological mechanisms during psychotic episodes that can also result in hyponatraemia. I will describe these mechanisms in chapter one. All that said, however, and while my book is primarily concerned with challenging the more standard kind of so-called 'Primary Polydipsia', I will have some suggestions to make in this book's concluding chapter as to how the idea of hypovolemic dehydration might actually have some surprising relevance for schizophrenia patients after all, at least in some cases. Whether my suggestions in this regard are worthy of further exploration is something for minds more expert than my own to judge.

There is something else that I should explain and which is on a different note to the rest of this introduction. In 2014-2015, I had a first round of ill-health in the form of POTS (Postural Orthostatic Tachycardia Syndrome), a condition that is closely related to ME/CFS and often overlaps with it. I recovered from POTS in 2015 by using a neuroplasti-city program, an experience which led me to write the book *POTS: What It Really Is & Why It Happens*. In that book, I suggested that a limbic system dysfunction was driving the condition and that this could be addressed using neuroplasticity. In late 2018, however, I developed ill-health again, this time primarily in the form of ME/CFS. My experience of illness this time has modified several of the views I put forward in my earlier book. I still think that there is merit in its general argument but would now regard the non-neurological complications of such illnesses as having at least equal weight as the neurological. I have published a correction on that book's website (www.whatpotsreallyis.net) in which I describe how my thinking has changed.

To return to the topic at hand and in conclusion to this introduction, I note that, in general, very few Primary Polydipsia researchers have ever questioned the assumptions that underly the condition. Those assumptions are simply assumed to be correct. There is a notable exception, however. In 2017, Prof. Daniel Bichet, Professor of Medicine at the Université of Montréal, wrote: 'The diagnosis of compulsive water drinking must be made with care and may represent our ignorance of yet undescribed pathophysiological mechanisms.'[5]

My work is just an hypothesis and I could, of course, be entirely wrong in my ideas. It is also possible that, even if I am right about hypovolemic thirst, this might still only represent one part of the so-called Primary Polydipsia puzzle and that other pathophysiological mechanisms may yet remain to be discovered in unravelling its mysteries. But, in general, I do hope, and strongly believe, that those 'yet undescribed pathophysiological mechanisms' are those of hypovolemic dehydration.

This book has four chapters in which I lay out my position.

In chapter one, I will consider the psychiatric origins of Primary Polydipsia and, in particular, the work of Barlow & De Wardener who, in 1959, wrote the most substantive early treatment of so-called 'compulsive water drinking'. I will then consider the current state of research into Primary Polydipsia: what have been the main developments and changes since the time of Barlow and De Wardener? In general, we will see that the legacy of those two authors lives on: some changes have occurred but these are generally unsubstantial and, in the main, thinking about the condition now is essentially the same as it was 60 years ago.

In chapter two, I shall describe the concept of 'Hypovolemic Dehydration' and explain how it can explain a polydipsia with a tendency towards very dilute urine and hyponatraemia. I shall then suggest that it is patients with ME/CFS, Long Covid and POTS (or 'Postural Orthostatic Tachycardia Syndrome', a condition closely related to ME/CFS and Long Covid) who are most likely to suffer from this kind of thirst, given

---

5. Bichet DG, 'The Posterior Pituitary' in Melmed S, Ed. *The Pituitary (4th Edition)*, 2017.

that hypovolemia is a common pathology within those conditions. As part of this, I shall explore the current research on low blood volume within these illnesses and theories as to why it occurs. Is it the excessive thirst within these conditions which has, at least in many cases, been historically misdiagnosed as 'psychogenic water drinking'?

In chapter three, I will mainly put my own voice aside and instead allow ME/CFS patients, and the doctors who treat them, to speak for themselves. This chapter is essentially a compilation of evidence regarding excessive thirst within ME/CFS, evidence which helps us to clarify its nature: what are the characteristics of this kind of thirst? And what kind of remedies have patients applied to improve it? Finally, we will consider some instances of where other ME/CFS patients have also been (mistakenly) diagnosed with Primary Polydipsia because of their thirst.

In chapter four, I will offer my own ideas regarding how to treat hypovolemic dehydration successfully, both in an acute (i.e. hyponatraemic) context and in terms of more general daily management. In this regard, I shall particularly recommend the drinking of Oral Rehydration Solution but I will also discuss other, more conventional medical options such as Flurinef, a synthetic form of the salt-retention hormone, aldosterone.

Finally, in the concluding chapter, I will consider possible objections to my hypothesis as well as its implications for two subsets within Primary Polydipsia, namely Dipsogenic Diabetes Insipidus and also the excessive thirst that can occur in some schizophrenic patients. I will also discuss how my ideas could be validated before offering some final remarks on the urgent need for rethinking the nature of so-called Primary Polydipsia.

And so, with all that said, I will now try to make my case.

Note 1: I welcome any correspondence about the ideas in this book. To write to the author, please use the contact form at: www.patrickussher.com

Note 2: The terms used to describe 'Primary Polydipsia' in the medical literature have been numerous and varied. I generally use 'psychogenic water drinking' and 'compulsive water drinking' and, in the context of my hypothesis, regard these as essentially interchangeable.

Chapter One

Freudianism and Primary Polydipsia - Past & Present

The early history of so-called psychogenic water drinking is somewhat obscure. Indeed, a PubMed search for 'psychogenic polydipsia' from 1900 to 1970 will yield only 26 results and a fair few of these papers are not even primarily concerned with the illness. It seems that the condition was first noted in 1905 by two French researchers, Ramond and Achard,[6] who used the term 'potomania' (from the Greek for 'water-madness'). From that point, various attempts to understand the condition were made but these were few in number. By far the most important and substantive early treatment of so-called Primary Polydipsia came from De Wardener, a kidney specialist, and Barlow, a psychiatrist, in 1959. Their paper, 'Compulsive Water Drinking', set out to analyse the cases of nine so-called compulsive water drinkers and will be the central focus of my discussion regarding psychiatry's early influence on the condition.

Barlow and De Wardener's work is important for three main reasons, each of which we will explore in this chapter.

---

6. As recorded by Cramer B., in 'La Potomanie' in Eds. Lebovici S. et al., *Nouveau traité de psychiatrie de l'enfant et de l'adolescent*, 2014, 1839-1842.

Firstly, it demonstrates such a strong bias towards psychologising the symptoms of so-called compulsive water drinkers that no objective reader could fail to question the assumptions which underlie the early thinking about Primary Polydipsia. Indeed, the amount of Freudianism[7] on display is almost parodic when viewed from the perspective of our own age and it would be impossible to imagine such a paper being written nowadays. This is all the more sobering when we consider that, in essence, the central physiological assumptions and diagnostic procedures regarding Primary Polydipsia are almost the exact same now as they were in Barlow and De Wardener's paper. Imagine if this scenario applied to a different illness, such as Type II Diabetes. If that illness had been assumed to be psychogenic by medical scientists back in the 1950s, and no one had ever challenged that assumption right up to the present day, and all of the current medical procedures, diagnostics, and so forth, were still by-products of that psychogenic worldview, would this not be an utterly ludicrous scenario? And yet this is precisely the situation with so-called Primary Polydipsia.

The second reason why a consideration of this paper is important relates to its necessarily limited understanding of thirst biomechanisms. In 1959, it was believed that the brain had only one thirst centre, the osmotic one, and there was no knowledge about the hypovolemic thirst centre at all: that was to come in the next decade. In this way, Barlow and De Wardener's paper suffers from a lack of essential physiological knowledge, knowledge that could have actually explained the central symptoms of so-called Primary Polydipsia from the beginning. Instead, as their work was limited to considering the problem purely through the

---

7. When I use the term 'Freudianism', I refer to the general tendency to suggest psychosomatic origins for a patient's symptoms, as if the latter were a manifestation of, for example, subconscious forces or intrapsychic conflicts. I do not strictly mean therefore everything pertaining to Freud's understanding of human psychology nor do I mean to dismiss certain observations he made that might clearly have some merit.

lens of osmotic thirst, a range of central assumptions regarding so-called Primary Polydipsia were developed, assumptions that have persisted as mainstays to this day. As such, Barlow and De Wardener attributed the purportedly psychological cause to the supposed significance of dilute urine in the context of hypo- rather than hypernatremia and the supposed importance of intact vasopressin function. Without a knowledge of hypovolemia-induced thirst, both intact vasopressin release and a hyponatraemic state point inevitably to a psychogenic cause. But what if these clinical features have always been framed incorrectly?

Finally, their paper is important for a third reason. For what were these nine patients really suffering from? When you strip the paper of its Freudian-esque jargon and consider more objectively the various symptoms these patients had, it seems quite clear that they were actually suffering from ME/CFS. This adds considerable weight to my general hypothesis that it is ME/CFS patients who have always been historically misdiagnosed as compulsive water drinkers because of a misreading of their hypovolemia-driven thirst.

Having explored the foundational thinking behind the initial concep-tualizations of Primary Polydipsia, we will then consider, in the second half of this chapter, the current state of the research regarding the condition. In doing so, we shall see that the most significant developments concern the emergence of various subtypes. In particular, experts nowadays tend to distinguish between so-called Primary Polydipsia as it might occur in psychiatric populations with severe mental ill-health, especially those with schizophrenia, and as it might occur in the general population (in which the majority of cases are to be found). We shall review specific mechanisms that have been identified within schizophrenic patients, mechanisms that can create hyponatraemia during psychotic episodes, although the initial reason for the polydipsic behaviour within schizo-phrenia remains unknown. Another significant change concerns the emergence of a subtype termed 'dipsogenic polydipsia' or 'dipsogenic diabetes insipidus', a condition in which it is thought that thirst-related defects drive the drinking although, again, the cause is unknown. In this chapter, I am not concerned with challenging these subtypes: I will offer some observations in this book's concluding chapter about how hypovolemic thirst could offer explanations for excessive thirst in the case of both of them, at least for some patients but, for now, I am merely concerned with describing the current understanding. Another significant development includes an additional diagnostic test for Primary Polydipsia, in the form of measuring copeptin, a compound far more stable than vasopressin and which acts as a kind of surrogate marker for it. But what we shall see is that, in general, nothing much has changed since the time of Barlow and De Wardener. The cause of Primary Polydipsia is still recognised as unknown, the behaviour of so-called Primary Polydiptics is still regarded as mysterious, and despite the acknowledgement of both of those things, something which should surely preclude any strong pronouncements as to its aetiology, the condition is still nevertheless generally described as being psychological and without physiological basis.

But before we turn to our discussion of Barlow and De Wardener, let us, as it were, set the scene by first considering briefly one of the earliest treatments of so-called psychogenic water drinking, namely the 1936 article *Psychogenic Factors in the Polyuria of Schizophrenia*, for this article gives us a clear sense of the early psychiatric bias that surrounded the condition. The author, Wilbur Miller MD, notes with approval the suggestion by an earlier psychoanalyst that polydipsia can signify a 'pre-Oedipus urethral fixation'[8] and, from this basis, he sets out to find 'factors in the personality and psychoses' among 12 particular patients who were drinking large amounts of fluid in the absence of any supposed physiological need. Wondering if the imbibing 'itself served as

8. 419.

a source of gratification or as a means of alleviating unpleasant tensions', Miller concludes that a striking feature of these patients is the 'failure of the group as a whole ever to have reached any degree of an adult heterosexual level of adjustment'. As part of this, he notes that 11 of the 12 patients had never shown 'any interest' in the opposite sex and that, in at least three cases, 'definite overt homosexual experiences' were (supposedly) causal in the development of their psychoses.[9] In general, Miller suggests that these patients are 'regressing' to a pre-adult state in which oral zones (i.e. the mouth) take on a subconscious erotic function. As these patients do not engage in normal heterosexual sex, they are instead imbibing large quantities of fluid as an 'oral method of libidinal gratification',[10] i.e. as some kind of subconscious surrogate activity for the sex they should really be having.

How would a modern day doctor react to learning that some of the earliest observers of so-called Primary Polydipsia were content to suggest that its symptoms stemmed from being gay? One would hope that it would make them think twice about the supposedly psychogenic basis of the whole condition. In any event, this paper is clearly not an example of the scientific method in action: it is rather the product of an old-school psychoanalytic worldview and filled with the assumptions and myths that underpin it. And yet this kind of worldview is precisely what formed and shaped the earliest impressions of this kind of polydipsia and it is a worldview that has never been successfully shaken off.

With this (rather unimpressive) backdrop now set, let us turn to consider the most thorough and influential of the earlier papers on psychogenic polydipsia, namely the aforementioned 1959 article 'Compulsive Water Drinking' by Barlow and De Wardener.

---

9. 423.

10. 426.

The Perspective of Barlow and De Wardener

Before we consider in detail their paper, we should discuss briefly the background of these two medical researchers.

Hugh de Wardener was, by all accounts, an exceptional medical physician. His work included breakthroughs in understanding the role of B1 deficiency in beri-beri as well as the causal effect of excessive sodium on the development of hypertension. He was also pivotal in the development of dialysis for patients with kidney dysfunction (indeed, he wrote a standard textbook entitled *The Kidney*) and was awarded an OBE for his contributions to medicine. In addition, he faced challenging circumstances in his life, including capture by the Japanese early in World War II after which he cared for the sick in Japanese prisoner of war camps until the end of the conflict.[11] Meanwhile, Erasmus Darwin Barlow[12] studied medicine at Cambridge and, while he went on to publish papers on physiology, his primary interest was in psychiatry. Indeed, he was senior lecturer and honorary consultant in psychological medicine at St Thomas's Hospital Medical School in London from 1951 to 1966. He was also the great-grandson of Charles Darwin.

Of these two, therefore, it seems likely that the psychiatric inter-pretation of (supposedly) psychogenic polydipsia owed more to the work of Barlow than to that of De Wardener.

In overview, the paper examines nine so-called compulsive water drinkers, considers aspects of their psychological state or development and makes various observations on the diagnostic procedures for distin-guishing between compulsive water drinking and Diabetes Insipidus. It ends with in-depth case studies of three of the patients.

11. This summary is taken from his 2013 obituary in *The Guardian*: https://www.theguardian.com/science/2013/oct/29/hugh-de-wardener

12. https://en.wikipedia.org/wiki/Erasmus_Darwin_Barlow

The paper, as noted above, is instructive for us in three main ways: i) the psychologization of the patients described and the complete absence of considering any alternative physiological explanation for their symptoms ii) its narrow attempt to understand the symptoms purely from within the lens of osmotic thirst physiology and its resultantly misguided assumptions about supposedly key clinical features, diagnostic procedures, and the like and iii) the fact that, when stripped of its psychiatric jargon, the patients in question were likely really suffering from ME/CFS.

Let us now consider each of these points in turn.

The Psychologization of 'Compulsive' Water Drinkers

It is striking that the possibility that the nine patients under question could be suffering from anything other than something psychological is never entertained. Instead, it is simply stated that: 'It is customary and reasonable to consider that compulsive water drinking occurs in emotionally disturbed people.'[13] Needless to say, this is not a scientific statement and speaks, if anything, to the fact that the supposed psychiatric cause of Primary Polydipsia has always been based on just that, namely supposition. In contrast, medical science requires hypotheses that can be proved empirically and not just 'customary' or 'reasonable' statements.

These kinds of assumptions are 'backed up' by an analysis of the patients' psychological history and characteristics. The authors write:

> 'Neurotic traits were common in childhood; a history of instability and vague illness during early years was obtained in all seven patients from whom a psychiatric history was obtained, and five of these had walked in their sleep. Schooling had often been interrupted, and adolescence had not been smooth. Work

---

13. 248.

histories, on the other hand, were very variable, and several patients had achieved positions of stability and responsibility, in spite of frequent interruptions through illness. All patients had had episodes of time off work through illness, or frequent or unexplained changes of work. No patient had a history of a stable and satisfactory sex life. Their difficulties included menstrual disturbances since puberty and many gynaecological operations (for example, patient No. 8, who also had premenstrual aphonia). Six patients had married; subsequently there had been many discordant and unhappy episodes...and separation in several cases. The patients had abstemious habits, except for a few who smoked heavily.'[14]

Freudianism abounds here: their childhoods were neurotic, their adolescence far from smooth, none of them had a satisfactory sex life, their marriages were troubled and they were in the main prudish types. That these things should have appeared so relevant to the authors, and not other factors, most likely speaks to their preconceived assumptions about the condition's cause. But why on earth should being 'abstemious' or a lack of sex be a relevant consideration? Being a celibate and sober individual might not be the most fun but it is, in and of itself, surely not guaranteed to lead to the desire to down 10 litres of water every day. Clearly, the authors here are not making use of the laws of medical physiology to make their case but are rather employing fashionable ideas of a Freudian nature, ideas which, however convincing they may have seemed to these authors, have never been proven empirically.

The psychosomatic interpretations continue. The cause of each patient's symptoms is attributed variously to 'conversion hysteria', 'delusional hypochondriasis' or 'depression'.[15] The health complaints of the patients are typically dismissed. For example, one patient

14. 235.

15. 242.

had episodes of 'paralysis' in the hospital but these are written off as 'functional'.[16] Another patient, having been treated with synthetic vasopressin as part of the study, then continued to drink enormous volumes of water, became dangerously hyponatraemic, vomited, developed incontinence and appeared to lose consciousness. Despite this rather serious state of affairs, the patient was then described by the authors, remorseless in their analysis even at such a moment, as developing 'hysterical fugue'.[17] Barlow and De Wardener were also keen to point out that, of all recorded case studies of patients with either compulsive water drinking or with Diabetes Insipidus, 79% of the former were women while, amongst the Diabetes Insipidus group (i.e. those with a 'real' illness), that figure dropped to 41%.[18]

Are modern medics aware that these kinds of ideas underpinned the early attempts to understand so-called Primary Polydipsia? I very much doubt it. My own hunch in this regard is that most doctors are simply unaware of the condition's history. They will assume that it must be a well-validated and researched condition. In medical school, they are not taught about Barlow's fondness for conversion disorders. They are simply taught that to diagnose Diabetes Insipidus, the following conditions need to be met, and to diagnose Primary Polydipsia, these requirements need to be met, and so on. The textbook says it is the case and therefore it is and if it is in the textbook, then surely the condition is well-founded. In contrast, I do believe that if doctors knew of the kind of suppositions which initially informed Primary Polydipsia, that they would simply be horrified to learn that they were unknowingly

---

16. 253.

17. 245-246. Dissociative fugue, formerly called fugue state or psychogenic fugue, is a subtype of dissociative amnesia. It involves loss of memory for personal autobiographical information combined with unexpected and sudden travel and sometimes setting up a new identity.

18. 247-248.

perpetuating such deeply unscientific ideas and ones associated with significant medical abuse, historically speaking.

Therefore, the first key point from considering Barlow and De Wardener's paper is to remember that they made use of ideas that are (or at least should be) anathema to modern medical practice. Regarding its supposed psychological basis, rigorous hypotheses were not developed or evaluated. Instead, 'reasonable' and 'customary' suppositions were made, suppositions that were primarily informed by trendy ideas of a Freudian nature. While the medical textbook might therefore state seemingly well-founded physiological observations about Primary Polydipsia, the worldview which created those observations shows us that, in truth, what the textbook has to say is merely built on sand.

Let us now turn to consider the second striking feature of Barlow and De Wardener's paper, namely its necessarily limited understanding of thirst physiology, an error that has also persisted unchallenged to the present day and with far-reaching consequences.

The Error of Situating Primary Polydipsia Purely in the Context of Osmotic Thirst Regulation

As we shall explore in more detail in the next chapter, this book's central thesis is that the symptoms of so-called Primary Polydipsia can all be explained in light of the hypovolemic thirst centre. However, it is important to remember that the hypovolemic thirst centre was not discovered until the 1960s,[19] long after the idea of Primary Polydipsia, and its supposedly psychiatric basis, was first conceived. Therefore, the knowledge of thirst physiology that informed the early understanding of so-called compulsive water drinking was necessarily limited. This limitation is essentially expressed in the central error that has always

---

19. Arai et al., 'Thirst in Critically Ill Patients: From Physiology to Sensation', 2013.

underpinned the thinking around Primary Polydipsia, namely confining the understanding of the condition purely to osmotic thirst.

As a result of this lens, certain assumptions are made by Barlow and De Wardener regarding what should be the key characteristics, defining clinical features and diagnostic aims relating to the condition, all of which have persisted essentially unquestioned to the present day. Consider the following extracts from their paper:

> 'Compulsive water drinking is usually distinguished from diabetes insipidus by testing the integrity of the neurohypophyseal system. The methods used include the response of the urine flow or concentration to fluid deprivation, intravenous nicotine, and hypertonic saline....'[20]

> 'The finding that plasma osmolality in compulsive water drinking is less than in normal subjects but that it is greater than normal in diabetes insipidus, has not previously been described; it is in accord with the basic difference between the two conditions. In compulsive water drinking the initial disturbance is excessive drinking, and polyuria is the normal response to expansion and dilution of body fluids. In diabetes insipidus the initial disturbance is polyuria, and the excessive drinking is a normal response to contraction and concentration of body fluids. It follows that in compulsive water drinking the plasma osmolality will tend to be low, whereas in diabetes insipidus it will tend to be high.'[21]

All of these supposedly key characteristics about Primary Polydipsia are the result of the erroneous belief that thirst is only ultimately about water. As a result, testing the body's capacity to release vasopressin (i.e. the neurohypophyseal system referred to above) is seen as essential to making the correct diagnosis as is distinguishing the condition from

---

20. 246.

21. 249.

Diabetes Insipidus, in which vasopressin release is often completely impaired. Similarly, the presence of dilute urine, low osmolality and hyponatraemia all purportedly speak to an initial disturbance stemming not from anything physiological but purely from the excessive 'psychological' drinking of fluids. For if quenching thirst is ultimately only about water, then being in a state of excessive free water should negate the need to drink further fluids. On this view, such drinking must therefore be psychologically-driven. But all of these ideas are based merely on assumptions which are rooted in ignorance. That ignorance is that, in general terms, thirst is only about water and osmotic thirst regulation and, if that is the be all and end all of thirst physiology, then truly nothing else can possibly explain what is occurring in so-called Primary Polydiptics other than mental illness.

The principal takeaway from this section, therefore, is that Primary Polydipsia was conceived at a time in which it was thought that the brain only had one thirst centre, namely the osmotic one, and that every aspect of the symptom presentation in Primary Polydipsia has been subsequently viewed in this light. This has made it impossible to consider any other physiological explanation for its various symptoms. In contrast, had the existence of the hypovolemic thirst centre been known at the time of Barlow and De Wardener's work, along with the existence of endogenously-created hypovolemic illnesses, then the symptoms of so-called Primary Polydipsia patients could have been understood differently from the beginning. The starting point would have been different and the resulting lens and models for understanding the condition would likewise have been different.

Let us now turn to the final salient aspect of this paper.

The patients in Barlow and De Wardener's study were most likely suffering from ME/CFS

While the current understanding of relevant aspects of the pathophysiology of ME/CFS will be explored in detail in the next chapter, it is worth noting for now that, when stripped of their strong Freudian overtones, the descriptions by Barlow and De Wardener of their patients strongly suggest that they were really suffering from that illness.

One can make this inference for two key reasons.

The first concerns the aetiology of the health problems these nine patients had. In some cases, these were triggered by specific physical or psychological traumas, including a husband's death,[22] being in a bomb scare or having multiple surgeries, including with severe complications.[23] In other cases, 'relapses were sometimes precipitated by domestic stress or by an acute illness.'[24] This is very much in accordance with the development of ME/CFS which is usually brought on by some kind of major stressor, most typically a viral illness, but any illness or traumatic event, broadly understood, can trigger the condition.

Secondly, while the self-reported symptoms of the patients in question are rarely the focus of the paper, where these are reported they are also highly reminiscent of ME/CFS. For example, one 57 year old woman 'had shortness of breath on exertion for five years,'[25] a symptom that is a classic hallmark of ME/CFS and the exercise intolerance that is characteristic of the condition. Similarly, a middle-aged man complained of 'aching everywhere' which is also typical of the central symptoms of 'Post-Exertional Malaise'.[26] At the end of the paper, there are three

---

22. 236.

23. 235, 253.

24. 236.

25. 253

26. 255.

in-depth case studies, all of which are suggestive of typical ME/CFS triggering events and symptoms. I will just outline the first of these here but the others are similar.

The patient in question ('Case Study A') was a 57 year old woman with a history of multiple surgeries, including removal of her left ovary and a pelvic tumour.[27] At age of 49 she had a vaginal hysterectomy which resulted in serious complications including, as Barlow and De Wardener note, 'parametritis, thrombophlebitis, a brain-stem thrombosis, and hysteria' (regarding the last 'symptom', I guess they just really didn't want to let the poor patient off the hook!). These and other traumas are highly suggestive of initiating events for ME/CFS. In addition to experiencing 'breathlessness upon exertion', she also had 'feelings of suffocation', which could potentially have been the air hunger that is typical of the low CO_2 levels in the illness[28] or the microclotting pathophysiology that has been identified more recently.[29] Later, and very much in accordance with the sensory disturbances that can occur in ME/CFS, her sense of taste, smell and vision became impaired and, as she put it, 'everything seemed darker'.[30] She was in and out of mental hospitals before being hospitalised under Barlow and De Wardener's care for her polydipsia. Finally, after discharge from hospital, Barlow and De Wardener commented on her subsequent 'hysterical weakness of the legs', which would also appear to be a rather Freudian-esque description of the exercise intolerance that is central to the pathophysiology of ME/CFS.

---

27. 253 ff.

28. Natelson et al., 'Physiological assessment of orthostatic intolerance in chronic fatigue syndrome', 2022.

29. Pretorius et al., 'The Occurrence of Hyperactivated Platelets and Fibrinaloid Microclots in Myalgic Encephalomyelitis/Chronic Fatigue Syndrome (ME/CFS)', 2022.

30. I note that, when I feel badly ill, everything also 'seems darker'. It is an unpleasant symptom and one which may be due to autonomic changes.

In general, one gets the strong impression that this patient, and all the patients, described in this paper were likely suffering from ME/CFS. Of course, one is only left to interpret 'hints' in this regard. The paper has its own clear bias and the medical understanding of ME/CFS at that time was practically zero. Nevertheless, when read in this light, the paper adds weight to the idea that, perhaps, what has always been thought of as Primary Polydipsia is actually a kind of polydipsia that has been central to ME/CFS and that it is patients with the latter illness that have generally been historically misdiagnosed as compulsive/psychogenic water drinkers.

We have now considered Barlow and De Wardener's paper in detail: its clear psychiatric bias, its necessarily limited understanding of thirst physiology (i.e. its ignorance of the as yet undiscovered hypovolemic thirst centre) and the possibility that the patients in question were actually suffering from ME/CFS. From our discussion, I think it fair to suggest that the initial thinking behind Primary Polydipsia does not speak to a condition with strong theoretical foundations. Nevertheless, this early model for Primary Polydipsia has essentially remained the dominant one right up to the present day, albeit with some more minor modifications and developments. So let us now turn to consider the current thinking about the condition and draw out the most relevant changes in relation to it. What exactly has changed over the course of the last six decades? And how do experts regard the condition today?

Primary Polydipsia in the Present Day

In coming to the general state of research into Primary Polydipsia today, there have been several recent papers, in particular by Sailer et al. ('Primary Polydipsia in the medical and psychiatric patient: characteristics, complications and therapy', 2017), and by Goldman and Ahmadi ('Primary Polydipsia: update', 2020), that provide helpful overviews of current thinking about the condition. Drawing on these papers, and particularly the one by Goldman and Ahmadi, I will present and reflect upon the most salient current differences from the time of Barlow and De Wardener. These differences particularly relate to the ways in which the condition is categorised. In addition, there have been two other key developments: the finding of psychosis-induced hyponatraemia within schizophrenia and of 'Dipsogenic Diabetes Insipidus'. The former is thought to involve pathophysiological mechanisms specific to psychotic states that result in low blood sodium while the latter involves drinking excessive fluids because of thirst-related defects.

Ultimately, however, these changes do not represent any significant breakthroughs in understanding the condition.

Indeed, as Sailer states, treatment options remain 'scarce'. Variable results have been obtained from patient education, biofeedback training and group therapy. In psychotic patients, certain drugs have had some success. In non-psychotic patients, there has been variable success with drugs such as the beta-blocker Propranolol but, in essence, the evidence for successful interventions with any particular medication is low. In general, it is thought that treatment plans are difficult to enforce due to the supposedly psychological basis for the condition. As Sailer writes: 'Voluntary reduction of water intake would be the ideal therapy for PP, however, it often fails due to non-compliance of the polydiptic patient who suffers from thirst and compulsive drinking behaviour.'

Similarly, as regards diagnostic procedures, not much has changed either from the time of Barlow and De Wardener. The water deprivation test remains, as Sailer says, the 'widely accepted gold standard'. The use of a hypertonic 2.5% saline infusion, something that was also used right back at the start of the condition's history, is likewise still sometimes employed. In this case, the aim is to increase osmotic pressure, thereby creating a state of internal dehydration and coaxing the brain into releasing vasopressin in order to dilute the situation. One more recently introduced measure is to test copeptin levels. Copeptin is secreted commensurately with vasopressin but, unlike the latter which degrades within minutes, it can remain stable in a test-tube for up to a week. It is therefore considered a reliable indicator of vasopressin levels.

Let us now turn to consider the first significant development, namely how Primary Polydipsia patients are currently considered to fall into one or other of two categories.

Overarching Categorisations

For Goldman and Ahmadi, patients generally fall into one of two central groupings, the first being patients with 'Severe mental illness (SMI) and neurodevelopmental disorders' and the second being those with 'Other psychiatric and medical conditions and the general population'. The former category can include patients with schizophrenia, schizoaffective disorder, bipolar disorder, psychotic depression, autism and intellectual disabilities while the latter includes patients with mental health conditions such as anxiety, depression, alcoholism, obsessive compulsive disorder, anorexia nervosa and, indeed, patients without any mental health condition at all. Others in the second category may have suffered from a traumatic brain injury, or another serious health issue, that resulted in the development of Primary Polydipsia (although, to my knowledge, the mechanisms by which a traumatic brain injury, for example, should lead to Primary Polydipsia have not been spelled out: certainly such a scenario is not suggestive of a primarily psychological issue).

In the case of both of these categories, Goldman and Ahmadi state that the excessive drinking generally stems from a psychological cause. However, upon closer inspection, it becomes difficult to maintain such a position.

For example, in the case of the group with severe mental illness, Goldman and Ahmadi reference work by Millson and by May respectively in support of their claim that drinking in this group is not driven by a biological thirst. Millson and May both conducted question-naire-based surveys of patients with severe mental ill health about the reasons for their excessive drinking ('Millson et al., 'A survey of patient attitudes toward self-induced water intoxication, 1992' and May DL., 'Patient perceptions of self-induced water intoxication', 1995). On the basis of that research, Goldman and Ahmadi suggest that delusional beliefs typically drive the water consumption in this group or that the behaviour can be a way of coping with anxiety. However, I read the research by Millson and May and found that it cannot actually support such claims. In the case of Millson's paper, 40% of respondents actually did state that thirst was one of their primary motivators while only 10% cited delusions. Meanwhile, May's questionnaire did not even include the option to cite thirst as a motivator in the first place: only psychologi-cal reasons were presented as possible answers. These were: 'Bored; to feel less nervous; something beyond control; to feel less sad; to escape; peps me up; get a high when drink; to cleanse my body; habit obtained from watching others; voices tell me to; drink to get attention.' Clearly, the 45 patient participants in that study did respond in the affirmative to many of these reasons but one cannot assume that thirst was not a motivator if they were never even offered that option. And if some of these patients do actually suffer from a significant thirst first and foremost, then why are they *really* drinking so much? Would this not instead suggest a biomedical abnormality? And, if that is the case, then the current supposed significance of having Primary Polydipsia along with severe mental illness, i.e. that the drinking is driven by delusional beliefs or by emotional coping mechanisms that themselves stem from that severe mental illness, completely falls apart. Rather, something else would have to be going on, at least in the case of those patients who do experience a significant thirst.

Similarly, within the second group, i.e. those among the general population and with other mental or medical health conditions, Goldman and Ahmadi also attribute a psychological origin to the drinking, despite the fact that, as they also acknowledge, patients in this category do tend to cite excessive thirst as their primary motivator. At some points, their analysis seems rather stretched in order to maintain the supposed psychological cause. For example, it is stated that 'compulsive water drinkers' are often heavy smokers, drinkers of alcohol, and exhibit eating disorders and that these co-existing behaviours connect the drinking to addiction and other "oral fixations", a suggestion that harks back to the more Freudian-esque characteristics of the earliest research into the condition. Could it really be the case that these patients, who simply say that they are thirsty, are drinking so much because of some kind of subconscious 'oral fixation'? How likely is that really? Goldman and Ahmadi further describe these patients as follows:

> 'Others with PP also exhibit changes in the physiologic regulation of water intake that are in many cases related to emotional or, at least non-homeostatic, influences on water balance... As previously mentioned, the increased thirst in anorexia nervosa may be compensating for low food intake and diminishing hunger. Eating and drinking are mechanistically inter-related and are markedly influenced by the same environmental and especially social contexts. In addition to substituting for hunger, drinking may be a particularly effective means of addressing other emotional states not only because of the pleasurable effects of fluid ingestion but because of the intense non-specific arousal induced by thirst. In addition, the marked renal excretory capacity for water limits the acute physiologic impact of the excess intake. These factors together may promote learning to substitute drinking for more appropriate coping responses, particularly in the presence of altered hippocampal and ventral striatal functioning.'

What are these ideas based on? Certainly not on asking the patients themselves: they just say that they are thirsty. Clearly, when one

41

considers such passages, the psychosomatic view of so-called Primary Polydipsia is still well and truly alive and the key evidence, i.e. what the patient actually reports, continues to be ignored.

In general, I believe that this way of categorising so-called Primary Polydipsia patients is problematic and for two reasons.

Firstly, if I am correct that hypovolemic dehydration is the real problem, then the current dichotomous categorisation will one day be rendered completely irrelevant. It is perfectly feasible that both a schizophrenic and someone without any comorbid mental health condition, severe or otherwise, could suffer from hypovolemic thirst, particularly if they both share an underlying hypovolemic illness. Such a scenario would forcibly collapse the supposed distinction between Primary Polydipsia among those with severe mental ill-health and those without. Indeed, if the concept of hypovolemic dehydration is validated one day, then the whole current way of categorising these patients will have to be profoundly reconsidered: how can you possibly categorise patients accurately if you do not know what they are actually suffering from?

Secondly, and even if we accept the general conception of Primary Polydipsia as a psychogenic illness, it is hard to understand the logic of the two categorisations. Are the patients in each group really so similar to each other as to merit being categorised together? The lived experience, and underlying pathologies, of someone with an intellectual disability is very different from that of someone with autism or schizophrenia (although of course some patients may suffer from several such conditions simultaneously). Why place patients with such contrasting conditions together? And can one really say, even if the water drinking were driven by purely psychogenic reasons, that someone with autism is drinking huge amounts of fluid for the same reasons as someone with schizophrenia? The same problem arises with the second category of patients, i.e. those with 'other psychiatric conditions and medical conditions and the general population'. Even if it were true that the drinking is driven primarily for psychogenic reasons, what could possibly be the psychological link between a Primary Polydipsia patient with obsessive compulsive disorder, another without any mental health condition at all and a third who developed the condition purely as a result of a traumatic brain injury? Whatever the link is, these patients are so different from one another that a psychological connection seems highly unlikely.

Given how disparate a group these patients are, it makes far more sense that the likely common connection between all of them will be the previously unconsidered pathophysiology of hypovolemic dehydration. Such a pathology could explain why such different patients, whether they have autism, anxiety, schizophrenia, an intellectual disability, no mental health condition at all, depression or the after-effects of a traumatic brain injury, can nevertheless all suffer from a polydipsia that produces the *same* central symptoms. Under this view, the shared feature among all of these patients is nothing to do with their psychological state but is rather an organic, hypovolemia-driven thirst. Of course, I am not suggesting that hypovolemic dehydration is the only cause of thirst in these groups: there may be other reasons for it. It could, however, provide a unifying explanation for the polydiptic behaviour among many of these patients, at least where physiological thirst is the primary motivator.

Let us now turn to consider the two other key developments since the time of Barlow and De Wardener, namely the finding of psychosis-induced hyponatraemia and of Dipsogenic Diabetes Insipidus.

Dipsogenic Diabetes Insipidus and Psychosis-induced Hyponatraemia in Schizophrenia

Dipsogenic Diabetes Insipidus (sometimes referred to as 'Dipsogenic Polydipsia') was first noted in the 1980s in studies by Mellinger and

Robertson respectively.[31] In this case, it is believed that some kind of neurological dysfunction has changed a patient's set point for experiencing thirst. In other words, their brain creates a real thirst signal long before the body's true osmotic needs. As a result, Dipsogenic Diabetes Insipidus is not considered to be caused by mental ill-health. The possible cause is unknown but it is thought that, at least in some cases, brain lesions can disrupt the normal thirst signalling pathways. We will return to this condition in this book's concluding chapter as I believe that, in the main, it can also be explained by my central hypothesis.

The second development concerns pathological mechanisms specific to schizophrenia (according to Sailer, Primary Polydipsia is observed in around 11-20% of schizophrenic patients). However, these pathological mechanisms do not explain the polydipsia itself – the cause of this is still regarded as unknown in schizophrenia – but they do explain possible mechanisms by which such patients might become more prone to hyponatraemia, at least during psychotic episodes. At such times, it seems that schizophrenic patients can suffer from increased neurological dysregulation, resulting in an inappropriate and excessive release of vasopressin. This is considered a form of SIADH (Syndrome of Inappropriate Anti-Diuretic Hormone) and essentially involves too much vasopressin release relative to the body's true physiological needs. As a result, too much water is retained and a dilutional hyponatraemia is created. In 1985, Vieweg was the first medical researcher to suggest that these kinds of mechanisms might be at play in schizophrenic patients[32] rather than something purely psychogenic. Later work by Goldman[33]

31. Mellinger, 'Primary polydipsia. Syndrome of inappropriate thirst', 1983 & Robertson, 'Dipsogenic diabetes insipidus: a newly recognized syndrome caused by a selective defect in the osmoregulation of thirst', 1987.

32. Vieweg, 'Psychogenic polydipsia and water intoxication - concepts that have failed', 1985.

33. Goldman et al., 'Psychotic exacerbations and enhanced vasopressin secretion in schizophrenic patients with hyponatraemia and polydipsia', 1997.

was instrumental in further clarifying this increased vasopressin during psychosis. Drawing on this research, Sailer writes: 'During acute psychotic episodes, worsening of polydiptic behaviour and increased levels of AVP (i.e. vasopressin) have been observed. It is speculated that during acute psychosis, the activation of the hypothalamic-pituitary-adrenal axis and AVP secretion influences behavioural traits and vice versa - probably through hippocampal involvement.'

These kinds of pathophysiological mechanisms would appear to be suggestive of a polydipsia specific to schizophrenia and, as I mentioned in the introduction, I am not primarily setting out to challenge this subset of Primary Polydipsia. On the face of it, my hypothesis does not tie in with a dysregulation that might increase vasopressin during a psychotic episode and, perhaps, this kind of Primary Polydipsia will always fall into its own category. That said, it is still theoretically possible that certain schizophrenics might suffer from an extreme thirst not because of something to do with schizophrenia *per se* but because they have a hypovolemic illness as a comorbidity. Furthermore, there may be reasons to think that at least some schizophrenics have more in common with patients with hypovolemic illnesses, like ME/CFS, than one might initially imagine. I will outline possibilities in this regard in the book's concluding chapter.

***

In reviewing the changes that have occurred in Primary Polydipsia over the last sixty years, with some minor exceptions, we can see that really, for the vast majority of so-called Primary Polydipsia patients, the situation remains roughly the same as it always was. The condition is still essentially considered a mystery. As Sailer writes: 'The pathogenesis of insatiable thirst and excessive fluid intake as seen in Primary Polydipsia remains largely unknown'. And, without knowledge of the cause, it is unsurprising that no successful treatments have been found and no real help is, as of yet, forthcoming for so-called Primary Polydipsia patients.

It is my contention that the supposedly 'mysterious' nature of the condition has stemmed from the mistaken lens through which its symptoms were first viewed, a lens that we have explored in the first part of this chapter. That early legacy, in which ideas of a Freudian nature were so prominent, resulted in viewing the condition in psychological terms, an assumption which, despite the fact that the cause is still acknowledged as unknown, has persisted ever since. At the same time, that early lens also framed the condition's symptoms in a purely osmotic framework, setting up a legacy by which the core assumptions and diagnostic procedures concerning the disorder have all remained confined to a very narrow physiological worldview. In order to break those shackles, fresh thinking is needed.

And so let us now turn to understand what might really be going on in so-called 'Primary Polydipsia'.

Chapter Two

Why Hypovolemic Dehydration Can Explain the Real Root Cause of 'Primary Polydipsia'

The central error in the understanding of Primary Polydipsia to date has stemmed from viewing the condition solely in relation to osmotic thirst physiology. If thirst is only, in general terms, about an excess or deficit of water, and all other known causes of thirst have been ruled out, then it makes no sense for someone to drink huge quantities of fluid. On this view, the only explanation for why someone might do so must be mental ill-health. Therefore, in order to challenge the current premise of Primary Polydipsia successfully, an alternative model that can explain its typical symptom presentation in organic terms is essential. It is the concept of hypovolemic dehydration that can provide this.

To start this chapter off, therefore, I will first describe the nature of the hypovolemic thirst centre. When is it triggered, how is it quenched and which bodily systems are involved? Then, we shall map out, in abstract terms, a model for a hypovolemic polydipsia driven by purely endogenous factors. In such a polydipsia, what kind of symptom presentation would one expect to see? I shall suggest that hypovolemic thirst, if mistakenly dealt with just by drinking pure water, will indeed result in clinical features that are the exact same as that which are observed in so-called 'Primary Polydipsia', i.e. overly dilute urine with a tendency towards hyponatraemia.

But if Primary Polydipsia has always really been hypovolemic dehydration by another name, then who, exactly, has been suffering from this hypovolemic thirst and why? I will argue that it is patients with ME/CFS who have generally been historically misdiagnosed as psychogenic water drinkers. I make this claim both because ME/CFS often involves a profound and endogenously-created hypovolemia and because ME/CFS patients often suffer from excessive thirst along with dilute urine and low blood sodium levels (this second aspect will be demonstrated in the next chapter). As many readers of this book will likely be unfamiliar with the condition, I will provide an overview of key research into the illness. Then, we will delve in detail into the hypovolemia that underpins the condition: just how short on blood are ME/CFS patients and what exactly does the research have to say on why this low blood volume is created? But I do not think that it is only ME/CFS patients who suffer from hypovolemic dehydration and, as such, we shall also consider other conditions which may include hypovolemic thirst, such as POTS and Long Covid (although both of these frequently overlap and share many mechanisms with ME/CFS). Finally, we shall consider how previous research into Primary Polydipsia, when looked at in a new light, may have been describing, all along and unknowingly, hypovolemic dehydration. Indeed, there are two papers in particular that, as we shall see, long ago identified that a suppression of blood volume retention hormones as well as a profound solute loss, for reasons entirely unrelated to the drinking of large amounts of water, seemed to occur in so-called 'Primary Polydipsia'. The real implications of those findings, however, were never explored.

Understanding Hypovolemic Thirst

The hypovolemic thirst centre was first discovered in the 1960s[34] and its central physiological role is entirely different from that of the osmotic thirst centre.

The key function of the hypovolemic thirst centre is to generate a thirst signal when the body experiences a significant drop in blood volume. This thirst centre is physiologically distinct from the osmotic thirst centre and has different functions. Arai et al. describe the differences between osmotic and hypovolemic thirst in the following extracts:

> 'Subtle changes in plasma osmolality are the most potent stimulus for (osmotic) thirst. In response to increases in osmolality, osmore-ceptors activate release of the neurohormone vasopressin (also known as antidiuretic hormone). The released vasopressin acts on the kidneys to conserve water to correct the hyperosmolar state. If this compensatory mechanism is unsuccessful, thirst arises to promote drinking. Thirst induced by marked volume loss, in contrast, is more closely related to the volemic and pressure changes regulated by the renin-angiotensin-aldosterone system.'

> 'Earlier studies suggested that increased extracellular plasma tonicity that resulted in cellular dehydration was the primary stimulus for thirst. Hypovolemia (i.e., an extracellular deficit) was not recognized as a stimulus of thirst until the 1960s.'

> 'Hypovolemic thirst mechanisms associated with changes in intra-vascular volume and pressure are less sensitive than are those associated with osmotic changes. For example, a decrease of approximately 10% of the plasma volume is required to initiate thirst, whereas only a minimal 1% to 2% increase in the plasma osmolality can stimulate thirst and drinking.'

---

34. Arai et al., 'Thirst in Critically Ill Patients: From Physiology to Sensation', 2013.

From these extracts, we can understand the central characteristics of hypovolemic thirst: it is triggered purely from the loss of extracellular fluid rather than intracellular fluid; the forces that primarily attempt to correct it stem from the renin-angiotensin-aldosterone axis (a hormonal axis that controls salt balance in the body) and *not* primarily from vasopressin-related neural circuitry; it is not as sensitive as osmotic thirst in that a significant plasma volume loss of 10% needs to have occurred before it is activated. The fact that hypovolemic thirst is triggered only after a 10% drop in plasma blood volume is particularly important for the hypothesis of this book as shall become clear when we come to discuss ME/CFS later in this chapter.

Arai et al. also list various reasons for hypovolemic thirst, all of which involve 'marked reductions in plasma volume', such as those that can occur from 'haemorrhage, vomiting, diarrhoea, sweating, and diuresis'. This is very much the standard view regarding causal factors for hypovolemic thirst, namely that these are more serious medical events that cause blood loss (e.g., haemorrhage) or the result of internal reactions to exogenous assaults on the body (e.g. vomiting induced by a stomach bug). What is not currently considered in standard thinking on hypovolemic thirst is that it might be induced as a result of an endogenous and self-maintained state of low blood volume. While such mechanisms exist in ME/CFS and POTS, these mechanisms are rarely taught more widely and, as such, the possibility of a kind of polydipsia driven by hypovolemic thirst has not yet been hypothesised.

Arai et al. go on to make another important point, namely that, in the case of hypovolemic thirst, drinking pure water can never suffice. Rather, hypovolemic thirst triggers 'sodium appetite' and requires appropriately concentrated fluids. They write: 'Sodium appetite refers to the sodium deficiency that occurs with the loss of extracellular fluids... the deficiency cannot be relieved solely by water intake without solute replacement...Correction of extracellular volume loss in hypovolemic hypotonic thirst requires replacement of both water and solute, mainly sodium.' Water alone can never quench hypovolemic thirst, no matter how much of it you drink. In order to boost plasma volume, the ingested fluids must be concentrated.

We have just considered the nature of hypovolemic thirst. Let us now consider how someone experiencing that thirst might actually develop symptoms that are exactly the same as those that are currently observed in so-called Primary Polydipsia.

Explaining 'Primary Polydipsia' with Reference to Hypovolemic Dehydration: A New Model

The following scenario illustrates how hypovolemic thirst can explain the typical symptom presentation observed in so-called Primary Polydipsia:

Imagine that, for purely endogenous reasons, someone experiences ongoing and significant solute loss, thereby leading to a chronic low blood volume of at least 10% less plasma than the physiological norm. Imagine further that those same endogenous reasons prevent the body from being able to resolve this hypovolemic state itself. As the plasma blood volume has dropped by at least 10%, the hypovolemic thirst centre, the body's last available means of correcting the deficit of blood, will activate, creating a strong thirst signal.

Naturally enough, the patient does not know that this thirst is not 'asking' for water but for appropriately concentrated fluids in order to boost blood volume. As a result, she just drinks water. But this water will, shortly afterwards, be urinated out: it is the physiological imperative of the kidneys to excrete water in a timely manner. Once this happens, the thirst will return as the quantity of blood remains low. In increasing desperation, the patient will continue to drink more water, only to find that nothing can ever quench her thirst. A vicious cycle of thirst and urination then begins, as the patient ingests more and more water, thereby producing ever more dilute urine.

As part of this model, hyponatraemia may develop for two reasons. Firstly, the endogenously-driven solute loss will push the body not only towards hypovolemia but also necessarily towards lower blood sodium levels. Secondly, the patient may drink so much because of their thirst that the amount of water creates an additional and dilutional form of hyponatraemia. This will only worsen the ongoing hypovolemia as salt, essential for blood's consistency and quantity, will also be washed out.

This model explains all the key features of so-called Primary Polydipsia: why excessive free water in the system does not quench the thirst (as the problem never concerned water but blood), why the urine becomes very dilute (as the patient erroneously keeps drinking a high volume of fluid to assuage their thirst) and why patients will go to desperate measures to consume fluid (as their body is experiencing a physiological emergency). This model also explains why vasopressin function being intact has no primary relevance for the patient's condition. Indeed, under this model, the endogenously-driven solute loss comes primarily from a suppression of the renin-angiotensin-aldosterone axis. We shall consider exactly how this suppression might occur later in this chapter but if this is where the real problem lies, then we can see how all current diagnostic procedures, which are concerned only with ascertaining the capabilities of osmotic-thirst related functions, are completely incapable of detecting the real problem. Finally, this new conception also suggests that the low blood sodium level is not created just from the sheer amount of ingested water, as is currently assumed, but also because of the endogenously-driven solute loss that starts the whole vicious cycle. This point is particularly important as it indicates that the hyponatraemia stems from an organic pathology rather than being purely the result of some kind of compulsion caused by mental illness. I will have more to say about this idea later in this chapter.

But for this potential model to be considered as plausible, we also need to identify a patient population which does suffer from endogenous low blood volume and which is also chronically thirsty. After all, endogenous hypovolemia is hardly likely to be a random occurrence but will rather come to exist via particular, illness-specific pathophysiological mechanisms. It is ME/CFS patients who are likely to fit this clinical picture, as we shall explore in detail shortly. Before that, however, let us first make some introductory remarks about the illness as it is possible that the reader of this book will be generally unfamiliar with the condition.

ME/CFS: An Overview

A central challenge to this book's thesis is that the vast majority of the medical profession is unaware of the research into ME/CFS. As a result, they may subscribe to the idea that it is a psychosomatic illness, a charge that has been levelled at ME/CFS patients consistently over the decades. I am not unaware of the problem of trying to counteract the idea that Primary Polydipsia is a psychosomatic illness by suggesting that it is actually driven by the symptoms of an illness that is often itself also considered psychosomatic.

However, those who view ME/CFS as a psychosomatic illness owe their position more to dogmatism than science. By this I mean that the idea ME/CFS is 'all in your head' is an assumption which dates from a time prior to the more recent research (particularly since the 1990s) which has been revealing a serious and multi-systemic pathophysiology. It is, in other words, an 'idée fixe' that has not caught up with what the research actually shows. While funding for the illness is still unacceptably low, enormous advances in understanding it have been made, including in understanding its core features of exercise intolerance and resulting episodes of 'post-exertional malaise' during which patients experience a temporary and significant worsening of symptoms. For example,

Harvard has identified cardiovascular abnormalities that are unique to ME/CFS. These are termed 'preload failure' and concern the poor venous return to the heart while orthostatic and are driven by autonomic changes, inappropriate arterial shunting and low blood volume among other dysfunctions.[35] Another possible reason for the exercise intolerance is the likely existence of 'microclots'. These tiny clots, visible under microscope, exist at a significantly higher rate in ME/CFS patients than in the healthy population.[36] They are capable of interfering with the transfer of oxygen from the bloodstream into the organs and muscles, thereby directly contributing to the lower anaerobic threshold within the illness and the post-exertional malaise. A research team in South Africa, led by Prof. Resia Pretorius, has developed a blood test for these microclots as standard clotting tests will not detect them. In addition, that ME/CFS patients have highly abnormal metabolic responses to exercise, relative to healthy but sedentary controls, has also been found in two-day exercise studies.[37] When we add in the existence of low blood volume, the pathophysiology of which we shall explore in detail shortly, we have a whole range of reasons for the reduced capacity to exercise that is so characteristic of the illness.

Research has identified other abnormalities too. For example, the research of Prof. Robert Naviaux at the University of California San Diego has found that, at a cellular level, the metabolism of ME/CFS patients is stuck in a 'Dauer' state.[38] This is a 'survival' state similar to that which is observed in starving animals. Stanford University, meanwhile, has its own ME/CFS research centre which is headed up by Prof. Ron Davis.

---

35. As summarised here: https://endmecfs.mgh.harvard.edu/heartpreload/

36. Pretorius et al., 'The Occurrence of Hyperactivated Platelets and Fibrinaloid Microclots in Myalgic Encephalomyelitis/Chronic Fatigue Syndrome (ME/CFS)', 2022.

37. Jin-lim et al., 'Prospects of the Two-Day Cardiopulmonary Exercise Test (CPET) in ME/CFS patients: A Meta-Analysis', 2020.

38. Naviaux et al., 'Metabolic features of chronic fatigue syndrome', 2016.

Work there has identified a likely biomarker for the illness, namely an abnormal cellular response to the stress of hypertonic saline.[39] There have also been abnormal findings in the brain (such as the shrinkage of certain areas, particularly to do with executive function and attention),[40] endocrine systems (for example, the adrenal glands of ME/CFS patients can shrink by up to 50%, likely contributing to hypo-adrenal output),[41] and the gut (such as dysbiosis)[42] as well as the identification of various autoimmune markers. Indeed, Prof. Carmen Scheibenbogen of Charité University Berlin, has been instrumental in finding these autoimmune components, in particular the presence of an excessive amount of Beta-2 Adrenergic autoantibodies.[43] These autoantibodies attach themselves to the blood vessels, preventing their normal vasodilatory capacities, leading to poor blood perfusion in the muscles (thereby providing another reason for the exercise intolerance) but also in the organs, including the brain. Indeed, along with her colleague Dr. Klaus Wirth, Prof. Scheibenbogen has published a trailblazing series of three papers that propose a model for the core pathophysiology within the illness. I will refer to these papers in the next section as they are central to understanding the low blood volume that is also so central to ME/CFS. For all the latest research on ME/CFS, I recommend the truly excellent

---

39. Davis et al., 'A nanoelectronics-blood-based diagnostic biomarker for myalgic encephalomyelitis/chronic fatigue syndrome (ME/CFS)', 2019.

40. Shan et al., 'Multimodal MRI of myalgic encephalomyelitis/chronic fatigue syndrome: a cross-sectional neuroimaging study toward its neuropathophysiology and diagnosis', 2022.

41. Scott et al., 'Small adrenal glands in chronic fatigue syndrome: a preliminary computer tomography study', 1999.

42. König et al., 'The Gut Microbiome in Myalgic Encephalomyelitis (ME)/Chronic Fatigue Syndrome (CFS)', 2021.

43. Scheibenbogen and Wirth, 'A Unifying Hypothesis of the Pathophysiology of Myalgic Encephalomyelitis/Chronic Fatigue Syndrome (ME/CFS): Recognitions from the finding of autoantibodies against ß2-adrenergic receptors', 2020.

blog, www.healthrising.org, run by Cort Johnson, an ME/CFS patient who writes summaries of the latest research findings in plain English.

I should also mention something that is usually underappreciated, namely the potential seriousness of ME/CFS. While some patients retain a reasonable level of functionality and can engage in full or part-time work and take some degree of normal exercise, an estimated 25% are either housebound or bed-ridden.[44] Of those in the last category, some patients can develop a very severe form of the illness, becoming completely bedbound and in need of ongoing care from family and/or medical professionals. Some of these patients cannot swallow and they receive nourishment intravenously or via a gastric tube. It is important to emphasise this point: the pathophysiology of ME/CFS is very serious and it can result in devastating consequences for the patient. Both from my own personal experience and having read of the experience of countless others, I am left at a loss regarding a world whose governments, doctors and often wider society do not care for the suffering of the profoundly sick in a way that would receive widespread condemnation if the situation concerned a different illness, such as cancer or MS.

In any event, it would be impossible for anyone to read the latest ME/CFS research and still be of the view that it is a psychosomatic illness. The problem is that the persistent notion that it is psychosomatic prevents physicians from giving the illness its due and taking the time to read the research in the first place. Most likely, they are unaware that this research is even happening. It is a bizarre thing that it is assumed that millions of people worldwide, all of whom complain of the same central symptom of devastating reactions to exercise (aka 'post-exertional malaise'), must all be simultaneously engaging in a hypochondrical pact. This, nevertheless, is an idea that many educated and otherwise smart doctors are happy to entertain. The almost systemic lack of

---

44. Davis et al., 'A Comprehensive Examination of Severely Ill ME/CFS Patients', 2021.

curiosity regarding the possible pathophysiology within the illness has backfired in recent times in particular with the emergence of Long Covid and the millions who suffer from it, most of whom have been left to their own devices. This is because, as we shall see later in this chapter, Long Covid and ME/CFS are essentially the same illness. Fortunately, there have always existed some doctors and medical researchers who believed their suffering patients and who have unravelled, bit by bit, many of the core mechanisms that drive the illness.

It is beyond the scope of this book to present all of the research that has been found in ME/CFS. I have given a short introduction above to some of its most recent and key findings so as to make clear that its pathophysiology is serious and that certain medical researchers at leading institutions around the world are engaged in ongoing investigations into it. For the purpose of this book, however, we do need to focus in depth on one particular aspect of the illness, namely the problem of low blood volume and the thirst that it potentially causes, as it is this which may hold the clue to unravelling the mystery of so-called Primary Polydipsia. And so let us now turn to consider how and why hypovolemia seems to occur in ME/CFS.

Low Blood Volume in ME/CFS

Under normal circumstances, a healthy human has around 5 litres of blood, of which plasma volume makes up 2.8 litres and red blood cell volume makes up 2.2 litres but, as we shall see, both of these amounts can drop significantly in ME/CFS. However, as with many illnesses, ME/CFS will not be experienced in the same way by every patient. In line with this, the research has largely clarified at this stage that, while there is a general trend towards hypovolemia in the illness, not all patients experience a significant drop in blood volume. That said there is, as we shall see, a subset of ME patients who do experience a profound hypovolemia.

So what has the research shown?

Early efforts at understanding this question resulted in a mixed picture, albeit one which clearly shows the presence of hypovolemia in the illness. For example, a 2000 study by Streeten et al. did find a significant reduction in RBC (Red Blood Cell) volume in 12 patients with ME/CFS when compared with healthy controls.[45] On the other hand, the same study did not find a significant difference in terms of plasma or total blood volume. A 2002 study by Farquhar at Harvard,[46] meanwhile, did find a trend towards lower blood volume in ME/CFS patients with a mean reduction in plasma volume of 9% compared with controls (in the same study, it was also found that the ME/CFS patients had 35% lower VO2 max, likely, at least in part, because of the cardiovascular strain that hypovolemia will create). In 2016, Newton et al. found no significant difference between the whole blood volume level in 41 ME patients and in 10 healthy controls but did find that 68% of ME patients had a RBC volume lower than 95% of the expected mean volume for healthy individuals. Similarly, in that study, 32% of patients also had a lower plasma volume than 95% of the expected mean volume for people in good health.

What emerges from these studies is the clear sense that lower blood volume affects some patients with ME/CFS more significantly than it does others. But why should this be the case?

One possible answer is illness severity. For example, a 2010 study by Hurwitz[47] et al. looked at 30 severe and 26 non-severe patients. In that study, the severe patients had only 57 ml/kg body-weight absolute

---

45. Streeten and Bell, 'The roles of orthostatic hypotension, orthostatic tachycardia, and subnormal erythrocyte volume in the pathogenesis of the chronic fatigue syndrome', 2000.

46. Farquhar et al., 'Blood volume and its relation to peak O(2) consumption and physical activity in patients with chronic fatigue', 2002.

47. Hurwitz et al., 'Chronic fatigue syndrome: illness severity, sedentary lifestyle, blood volume and evidence of diminished cardiac function', 2010.

blood volume (the healthy norm is around 65-70 ml/kg). On the other hand, the mean absolute blood volume for non-severe patients was 61 ml/kg, suggesting a clear correlation between the total amount of blood volume and how badly each patient is affected. However, while it makes sense that more hypovolemic patients should also be more severely ill, Hurwitz' study did not indicate which pathological features might lead ME/CFS patients into a more serious or alternatively a more minor form of hypovolemia.

A much clearer answer to the question of which ME/CFS patients experience a more profound kind of hypovolemia has emerged from the work of Visser and Van Campen in the Netherlands. In their 2018 paper 'Blood Volume Status in Patients with Chronic Fatigue Syndrome: Relation to Complaints', they looked at the presence of hypovolemia in ME patients with orthostatic intolerance and without. Orthostatic intolerance refers to a dysfunctional response to the challenges of being upright, typically driven by autonomic and cardiovascular changes (cf. the 'preload failure' identified by Harvard above), and which tends to be a primary contributor to exercise intolerance. What Visser and Van Campen found is that patients with orthostatic intolerance had significantly lower total blood volume than patients without it.

As this is the study best placed to clarify the subset of ME/CFS patients that is most relevant for the thesis of this book, let us consider it in more detail.

The study consisted of 11 female patients with ME/CFS. These patients underwent the 'standard dual isotope erythrocyte labelling technique' to determine blood volume. Overall results were expressed as absolute values (i.e. total and per kg body weight) and also as percentage normalized volume for total blood, red blood cell and plasma (i.e. the percentage given indicates the quantity of blood relative to the physiological norm). Four of the patients did not have orthostatic intolerance and seven of them did. Importantly, the seven with orthostatic intolerance were all housebound while the four without orthostatic intolerance were not, indicating that this is a key factor that predicts illness severity.

The results were striking. Patients without orthostatic intolerance had a total blood volume of 66 ± 9 (ml/kg) and 94% ± 10% normalised total blood volume. In patients with orthostatic intolerance, however, these numbers dropped profoundly. Their total blood volume was 55 ± 4 (ml/kg) and their total blood volume relative to the physiological norm was 77% ± 7%. A similar and also significant drop was seen in RBC and plasma volume between the two groups.

This finding casts the results from previous studies in a new light as those studies did not categorise their patients according to the presence or absence of orthostatic intolerance. Rather, with the exception of Hurwitz' study which divided patients into severe and non-severe, they generally presented their results as if their patients belonged to one homogenous group. To present the mean blood volume levels of a patient group that is compromised both of patients who are majorly hypovolemic and patients who are more minorly hypovolemic is something that cannot represent the true picture. In this way, the earlier results were somewhat skewed towards presenting a misleadingly 'middling' picture of how hypovolemia can play out in the illness. The fact is that there are ME/CFS patients who experience a profound hypovolemia and there are those who do not. When we look only at the former group, as Visser and Van Campen have done, we can see that the drop in blood volume for these patients is physiologically catastrophic. Similarly, as noted above, the severe patients in Hurwitz' study also had a blood volume level (at 57 ml/kg) which is essentially the same as the 55±4 (ml/kg) among patients with orthostatic intolerance in Visser and Van Campen's study. It is reasonable to assume, therefore, that ME/CFS patients with orthostatic intolerance and related low blood volume tend to have the severest forms of the illness and vice versa.

In this section, we have so far seen how the research has teased out the existence of a subgroup of ME/CFS patients who are profoundly hypovolemic. What this research does not indicate, however, is *why* these patients should have such low blood volume in the first place. Before we turn to consider that question, however, it is worth pausing at this point to reflect on how this subset of ME/CFS patients with low blood volume can fit into the overall thesis of this book.

In order to do so, let us remind ourselves of the reduction in blood experienced by the hypovolemic patients with orthostatic intolerance in Visser and Van Campen's study. The study's results indicate that the percentage normalised blood volume among this group is 77% ±7%. This means that the mean percentage of blood relative to the physiological norm is 77% but that the most hypovolemic patient with orthostatic intolerance had only 70% of the physiological norm while, at the other end, the least hypovolemic patient had 84% of the norm. Put another way, the mean reduction in blood volume from the physiological norm was 23%, the biggest drop was 30% and the lowest was 16%. Put in even more comprehensible terms, if a healthy human being has around 5 litres of blood, then, if we take this study as representative, the least hypovolemic patient (with orthostatic intolerance) had 4.2 litres of blood, the mean reduction resulted in 3.85 litres and the most hypovolemic patient had only 3.5 litres.

Earlier in the book, I mentioned that the hypovolemic thirst centre is triggered when plasma blood volume drops by 10%. What is apparent therefore is that, regardless of why this low blood volume comes about, these more severely ill ME/CFS patients are clearly in a situation in which *the threshold for the triggering of the hypovolemic thirst centre has long been passed*. Therefore, if it is accurate to suggest that hypovolemic dehydration could be a previously unappreciated and unmapped out kind of polydipsia, it is reasonable to assume that ME/CFS patients with orthostatic intolerance are *the* prime candidates for experiencing it.

In other words, we have both a potential model for how hypovolemic dehydration might create a polydipsia with a tendency towards dilute urine and hyponatraemia and we have a patient population to whom this model can obviously apply.

But why is this hypovolemia happening in the first place? Before we proceed to consider that question in detail, we should first make clear that it is *not* primarily caused by simple deconditioning. Indeed, some academics have liked to suggest that ME/CFS patients might be hypovolemic primarily because of the reduced cardiac output that deconditioning can cause. Under this view, the low blood volume might simply stem from extended bedrest and the supposed 'false illness beliefs' or 'exercise phobias' that some have bizarrely liked to suggest are behind the generally supine 'behaviour' of ME/CFS patients. However, research, also by Visser and Van Campen,[48] has demonstrated that orthostatic intolerance (which, as we have just seen, is the central predictor of hypovolemic severity in the illness) in ME/CFS is not caused by deconditioning. In a study which looked at orthostatic intolerance in both conditioned and deconditioned ME/CFS patients (for it is possible to have ME/CFS and still be relatively fit), no significant difference was found between the groups in terms of cerebral blood flow. Indeed, even fit ME/CFS patients had a reduction in cerebral blood flow similar to that which was observed in the most severely deconditioned patients. While deconditioning can of course contribute somewhat to a hypovolemic state as a result of a reduction in cardiac strength and can also contribute to a worsening of the quality of life of ME/CFS patients, the primary mechanisms in the illness are clearly the real culprit for the reduction in blood volume. If it were otherwise, then patients with other disabling conditions, conditions which might result in wheelchair use for example,

---

48. Visser and Van Campen, 'Deconditioning does not explain orthostatic intolerance in ME/CFS (myalgic encephalomyelitis/chronic fatigue syndrome)', 2021.

would also necessarily suffer from similarly profound reductions in blood volume but this is not something that has been observed.

And so let us now delve deeper into low blood volume in ME/CFS. How does someone's body, as a result of purely endogenous reasons, end up with such a shortfall of blood? We will examine this question from two angles. The first will be to consider why plasma volume in particular becomes lower in ME/CFS and the second will be to consider why red blood cell volume becomes lower. For, as we have seen from our discussion so far, both blood 'compartments' tend to be diminished in the illness, contributing to the overall hypovolemic state.

Plasma Volume Reduction: ME/CFS and The Renin-Angiotensin-Aldosterone 'Paradox'

The RAA axis (Renin-Angiotensin-Aldosterone axis) is a complex endocrine/neurohormonal system that controls salt balance in the body. Indeed, all three hormones, and in particular aldosterone, can retain salt and therefore plasma. Furthermore, the RAA axis also has a role in stimulating the release of vasopressin (antidiuretic hormone), although this, and all these hormones, are ultimately controlled by very complex, often interlinking, systems within the body. Textbooks will teach that, in a hypovolemic state, the body kicks the RAA axis into action in order to reabsorb sodium and boost blood volume. Arai et al. describe the standard progression of RAA axis activity in this regard as follows:

> 'In instances of progressively decreasing cardiac output (i.e., haemorrhage or extracellular dehydration), the kidneys are stimulated to release renin. Renin transforms the plasma protein angiotensinogen into the relatively inactive angiotensin I, which subsequently is catalysed by angiotensin-converting enzyme in the lungs into renal angiotensin II. The highly active angiotensin II causes vasoconstriction and acts directly on the sodium appetite centers. Released aldosterone, in turn, increases the

reabsorption of sodium in the kidneys to mediate hypovolemic thirst by increasing body fluid retention and osmolality to restore plasma volume.'[49]

What most medics are unaware of, however, is that these kinds of mechanisms do not work properly in ME/CFS. This is what is known as the RAA 'paradox' in ME/CFS research. Due to this suppression of the RAA axis, ME/CFS patients lose a considerable amount of salt in their urine. A basic rule of physiology is that water follows salt and so this solute loss will also lower plasma volume significantly. As a result, over time, a chronic state of low blood volume develops and, due to the very same RAA axis downregulation that created it in the first place, the body is also incapable of reversing the situation.

But why does this suppression of the RAA axis occur?

A first possible answer to this question emerges from the work of Miwa in Japan. In his 2016 paper ('Down-regulation of renin-aldosterone and antidiuretic hormone systems in patients with myalgic encephalomyelitis/chronic fatigue syndrome'), Miwa suggests that changes in the nervous system may account for diminished RAA axis activity and, therefore, for the hypovolemia.

The study, in which importantly all 18 ME patients also had orthostatic intolerance, set out to find the following factors:

'In the present study, cardiac function was echocardiographically determined and blood levels of the neurohumoral factors including plasma renin enzymatic activity (PRA) and concentrations of aldosterone and antidiuretic hormone (ADH), the main regulatory factors for circulatory blood volume, were determined in patients with ME as compared with those in healthy controls.'

As for the results, plasma renin activity, aldosterone and antidiuretic hormone were all significantly lower in ME patients than in controls, a

---

49. Arai, 'Thirst in Critically Ill Patients: From Physiology to Sensation', 2013.

finding that is particularly striking given that, in hypovolemic states, all of these hormones would be expected to increase significantly. The data were as follows:

Plasma Renin Activity (ng/ml/h) – Healthy Controls: 2.5 ± 1.5 ; ME/CFS Patients: 1.6 ± 1.0

Plasma aldosterone (pg/ml) – Healthy Controls: 157 ± 67; ME/CFS Patients: 104 ± 37

Antidiuretic Hormone (pg/ml) – Healthy Controls: 3.3 ± 1.5; ME/CFS Patients: 2.2 ± 1.0

Miwa suggests that this downregulation may be occurring because of changes in nervous system function, in particular as a result of Hypothalamus-Pituitary-Adrenal (HPA) axis impairment. In other words, under this view, the hormonal suppression is ultimately the result of a 'signalling problem'. Given that HPA axis problems have been identified in ME/CFS,[50] this hypothesis is quite likely to be at least partially true, although we also know, as mentioned earlier in this chapter, that the adrenal glands themselves can shrink by up to 50% in ME/CFS, which may theoretically decrease aldosterone output even further.[51]

However, a range of recent papers by two German researchers, Prof. Carmen Scheibenbogen and Dr. Klaus Wirth, offer another compelling hypothesis for the downregulation of the RAA axis in ME/CFS. In a series of three papers, Wirth & Scheibenbogen posit a convincing 'big picture' thesis for the whole pathophysiology of ME/CFS, from the brain, to the endocrine, cardiac and vascular systems, right down to sodium-potassium pump cellular exchange. Their work could represent the most

---

50. Tomas et al., 'A Review of Hypothalamic-Pituitary-Adrenal Axis Function in Chronic Fatigue Syndrome', 2013.

51. Scott et al., 'Small adrenal glands in chronic fatigue syndrome: a preliminary computer tomography study', 1999.

dramatic breakthrough in ME/CFS research to date and is essential reading for anyone interested in understanding the complexities of the illness.[52,53,54] I will not focus on all of their ideas here but will limit my discussion to their views on the RAA axis suppression within the illness.

In essence, Wirth & Scheibenbogen believe that central to the illness' pathophysiology is both a chronic vasoconstrictive state and a chronic impairment among vasodilatory functions. This situation is caused by autonomic changes (in the form of excessive sympathetic tone) and Beta2-adrenergic autoantibodies, both of which lead to the diminished functionality of Beta2-adrenergic receptors, which are particularly responsible for vasodilation. The result of this is poor blood perfusion and systemic hypoxia in the organs and musculoskeletal systems. As normal vasodilatory function is impaired, the body tries to rectify this state of affairs by enlisting emergency 'back up' vasodilatory systems, primarily through the activation of the KKS (Kallikrein-Kinin-System) and the release of bradykinin, a powerful vasodilator. While the activation of the KKS represents the body's attempt to rectify the chronic hypoperfusion, it comes with its own serious side-effects. In particular: i) the vasodilators are powerful enough to cause vascular microleaks leading to the transfer of extracellular fluid into the interstitial space and ii) as the KKS system naturally opposes the actions of the RAA axis, it downregulates the latter thereby increasing salt and water excretion. Under this hypothesis, we therefore have two possible reasons for the emergence of a hypovolemic state in ME/CFS: the actual leaking of blood from extracellular fluid into the interstitial space and an explanation for

52. Scheibenbogen and Wirth, 'A Unifying Hypothesis of the Pathophysiology of Myalgic Encephalomyelitis/Chronic Fatigue Syndrome (ME/CFS): Recognitions from the finding of autoantibodies against ß2-adrenergic receptors', 2020.

53. Scheibenbogen and Wirth, 'Pathophysiology of skeletal muscle disturbances in Myalgic Encephalomyelitis/Chronic Fatigue Syndrome (ME/CFS)', 2021.

54. Scheibenbogen, Wirth and Paul, 'An attempt to explain the neurological symptoms of Myalgic Encephalomyelitis/Chronic Fatigue Syndrome', 2021.

the significant blunting of the normal RAA axis response to preserve adequate salt & water balance. From the second of these, therefore, we have a compelling potential explanation for the RAA axis downregulation that has so perplexed ME/CFS researchers. It is particularly important to note that, for Scheibenbogen and Wirth, this RAA axis downregulation will become even more pronounced during episodes of post-exertional malaise during which all of the central mechanisms within the illness will necessarily flare up. This episodic deterioration can also explain why ME/CFS patients often note that their thirst is at its worst during periods of post-exertional malaise, as during those times solute loss will increase.

Personally, I believe elements of the hypotheses put forward by both Miwa and by Wirth & Scheibenbogen are likely to be correct. Only time will provide us with a complete answer to the question of the RAA-axis 'paradox' within the illness but what we do know for certain is that RAA axis suppression is central to the illness and a primary driver of the hypovolemia that usually accompanies it. And, assuming my general thesis is correct, this RAA axis suppression is clearly therefore the central driver of hypovolemic thirst and the real physiological initiator of the symptoms observed in what is currently termed Primary Polydipsia. From this perspective, we can see how the supposed importance of testing vasopressin function in so-called Primary Polydipsia patients has largely been a red herring: their actual issue has likely stemmed from elsewhere.

We have now discussed why plasma volume is reduced in ME/CFS but what about red blood cell volume? In this case, the possible answer is far more straightforward and actually probably linked to our preceding discussion about the diminished RAA axis activity.

Lowered Red Blood Cell Volume: Diminished Erythropoietin Production

As we have seen from the discussion of the studies by Newton et al. and by Visser and Van Campen, ME/CFS patients often have lowered red blood cell volume as well as lowered plasma volume. The question as to why this is the case has not received too much attention. However, the hormone erythropoietin (EPO), produced within the kidney, both protects red blood cells from destruction and stimulates the stem cells within the bone marrow to produce new red blood cells. As a recent study ('Effects of Angiotensin II on Erythropoietin Production in the Kidney and Liver') by Yasuoka et al. demonstrated, there appears to be feedback mechanisms by which the RAA axis regulates erythropoietin production to a significant extent. In that study, the administration of Angiotensin II stimulated erythropoietin production such that the authors concluded: 'These data support the regulation of EPO production in the kidney by the renin-angiotensin-aldosterone system (RAS)'. In line with this finding, it seems reasonable therefore to suggest that the hypovolemia stemming from lowered red blood cell volume ultimately stems from the same mechanisms as those which govern the diminution of plasma volume within the illness: as RAA axis activity becomes significantly diminished so too will there be a lowering of erythropoietin levels and, as a result, of red blood cell volume.

All in all, then, we have observed several possible key reasons for the lowered blood volume in ME/CFS of which RAA axis suppression leading to increased solute loss seems to be the most relevant. That RAA axis suppression appears to be driven either by the upregulation of the KKS system, a system which is antagonistic to the RAA axis, or by nervous system dysregulation or by a combination of both. In addition, we have seen both how the vascular microleaks might also contribute to the hypovolemia and how the RAA axis suppression likely not only decreases plasma volume but may incidentally reduce red blood cell volume as well.

I will just briefly mention two further thoughts of my own in relation to possible additional contributing factors to the hypovolemia within ME/CFS. Firstly, as mentioned in relation to the work of Pretorius et al., microclotting has been observed in ME/CFS at high levels. This will reduce the peripheral microcirculation and, therefore, the overall available 'space' for the body's blood. It is conceivable, therefore, that this also has its role to play, albeit a more minor one, in creating and maintaining the overall hypovolemia. Secondly, during episodes of post-exertional malaise, there is an excessive build-up of lactic acid and a disruption in the body's normal acid base. The kidneys, in an effort to avoid PH dysregulation, will work hard to excrete this lactic acid. As part of this necessary 'mop up' job, however, it is possible for various electrolyte disturbances to occur, including the loss of more sodium than might be excreted than under normal, healthy conditions.[55] Both of these last factors are more speculative but could feasibly worsen the general hypovolemic state within the illness.

As a result of all the aforementioned reasons, we can see how a profound hypovolemia can develop within ME/CFS and how, as a result, excessive thirst can be created due to the triggering of the hypovolemic thirst mechanism. And, as these dysfunctions all concern salt loss and resultant lowered blood levels, we can see how the understandably clueless patient, in their desperation to quench their thirst by drinking water, will never be able to resolve the thirst they experience, entering a vicious cycle which will look just like (and in fact be exactly the same as) that which is observed in so-called Primary Polydipsia.

We have now considered, in detail, how and why hypovolemia seems to occur in ME/CFS. But is endogenous hypovolemia only a feature

---

55. DiNicolantonio & O'Keefe, 'Low-grade metabolic acidosis as a driver of chronic disease: a 21st century public health crisis', 2021.

of that illness? Or could other illnesses also be capable of producing hypovolemic thirst?

Low Blood Volume in POTS & Long Covid

So far our discussion has suggested that hypovolemic thirst might be a natural outcome of the hypovolemia within ME/CFS. However, it is also feasible that any condition with endogenous hypovolemia might create such a symptom. One other prominent candidate is POTS (Postural Orthostatic Tachycardia Syndrome) in which some, though not all, patients also tend to have low blood volume. However, for those unfamiliar with POTS or with ME/CFS, it is important to mention that there is a significant overlap between these conditions, both of which are often described as being forms of 'dysautonomia'. Many POTS patients have ME/CFS and vice versa. They both belong to the same umbrella of illnesses which often tend to co-exist in affected patients, illnesses such as: MCAS (Mast Cell Activation Syndrome), hEDS (hypermobile Ehlers Danlos Syndrome) and FM (Fibromyalgia). A general review of treatment options for POTS and current research into the condition[56] included results from a survey of 3933 POTS patients regarding their co-morbidities. Of these, 25% had hEDS, 21% had ME/CFS and 20% had FM. As Vermino et al. note in that paper: 'A variety of other clinical diagnoses may coexist with POTS, but it is largely unclear whether the presence of one of these other diagnoses defines a unique pathophysiological subset of POTS. Patients with POTS may simultaneously meet the diagnostic criteria for migraine, hypermobile Ehlers-Danlos syndrome (hEDS), mast cell activation syndrome (MCAS) or chronic fatigue syndrome (CFS).' There are clearly commonalities that exist in this general cluster of illnesses and, as such, the following discussion of hypovolemia in POTS comes with the caveat

56. Vermino et al., 'Postural orthostatic tachycardia syndrome (POTS): State of the science and clinical care from a 2019 National Institutes of Health Expert Consensus Meeting – Part 1', 2021.

that I may simply be describing further aspects, or essentially the same aspects, of hypovolemia as found within ME/CFS.

In any event, how many POTS patients tend to have low blood volume? In their review of the current state of scientific research, Vermino et al. write the following:

> 'Absolute hypovolemia is commonly observed in POTS, with up to 70% of patients exhibiting deficits in plasma volume and red blood cell volume. This hypovolemia can reduce stroke volume and lead to compensatory tachycardia to maintain cardiac output and BP. The importance of hypovolemia in POTS pathophysiology is illustrated by the finding that some patients have reduced orthostatic tachycardia and improved symptoms after acute plasma volume expansion (e.g. intravenous saline, the vasopressin analog Desmopressin, exercise training). Ongoing studies are examining the impact of increasing plasma volume with dietary sodium, chronic intravenous saline, or albumin infusions in POTS.'

Why is the hypovolemia happening? Most interestingly, the likely central reasons for this hypovolemia stem from an RAA axis 'paradox', just as in ME/CFS. This is brought out in Raj et al.'s 2005 paper 'Renin-Aldosterone paradox and perturbed blood volume regulation underlying postural tachycardia syndrome'. This paper found that the overall total blood volume reduction in POTS patients, when compared to the ideal quantity, was 16.5% ± 6.8%, a finding which, as we have seen above, is very similar to that which was observed by Visser and Van Campen in ME/CFS patients. Despite this blood volume deficit, however, RAA activity remains suppressed. As Raj et al. write:

> 'Given their degree of hypovolemia, however, one would expect both plasma renin activity and aldosterone levels to be significantly higher in the POTS group than in controls. Both the plasma renin activity and, to a greater extent, aldosterone levels were inappropriately low given the hypovolemic status of the patients

with POTS. We have termed this dysregulation of plasma renin activity and aldosterone in POTS the "renin-aldosterone paradox."'

Raj et al. continue as follows:

'Aldosterone secretion is controlled at many levels: it is stimulated by angiotensin II, potassium, and hyponatremia, and acutely by the adrenocorticotropic hormone; it is inhibited by dopamine and atrial natriuretic factor (ANF). Electrolyte abnormalities are not likely to explain the low aldosterone as the sodium and potassium levels were similar in the POTS group and controls. Although we cannot exclude the possibility that there are abnormalities in ANF or increases in adrenal dopamine concentrations that could contribute to the low aldosterone state, the most likely explanation for the renin-aldosterone paradox is an inappropriately low level of angiotensin II.'

This speaks precisely to the RAA 'paradox'. In a hypovolemic state, angiotensin II should be high but, for whatever reason, its activity remains suppressed. Interestingly and on a personal note, when I tested my own angiotensin II level in the summer of 2021, it was found to be 11 (normal range: 19-38).

In addition, Raj et al. also propose various mechanisms by which red blood cell volume may become lower in POTS, mechanisms that are also similar to those which we discussed in the last section in relation to lower RBC volume in ME/CFS. The authors suggest that the lowered RBC volume in POTS may be explained either because of a close relationship between RAA axis function and erythropoietin production or because the body chooses to lower RBC volume so as to retain an appropriate level of haematocrit for the current level of plasma volume, a possible example of a necessary adaptation to a physiologically debilitating state of affairs.

In any event, given the significant reduction in blood volume that POTS patients often experience, it is likely that they could also suffer from a hypovolemic polydipsia and that these patients should also be included in any future research that might try to validate the idea of hypovolemic thirst. However, as I stated above, there are also significant overlaps, in terms of shared pathophysiologies, between POTS and ME/CFS. It is sometimes hard to say where one condition ends and the other begins. As such, while my book has tended to emphasise ME/CFS, its argument applies also to POTS and really to any other condition which may involve endogenously created and maintained hypovolemia.

One other such condition is, of course, 'Long Covid' although this also shares strong similarities with ME/CFS. Indeed, both the post-viral nature of the condition and the very similar symptom presentation have led researchers to suggest that Long Covid and ME/CFS may be essentially the same illness. For example, Visser and Van Campen in their 2022 paper ('Orthostatic Intolerance in Long-Haul COVID after SARS-CoV-2: A Case-Control Comparison with Post-EBV and Insidious-Onset Myalgic Encephalomyelitis/Chronic Fatigue Syndrome Patients') conclude as follows: 'OI (orthostatic intolerance) symptomatology and objective abnormalities of OI (abnormal cerebral blood flow and cardiac index reduction during tilt testing) are comparable to those in ME/CFS patients. It indicates that long-haul COVID is essentially the same disease as ME/CFS.' Similarly, a 2021 study by Dani et al.[57] suggested that 'long Covid' can be explained by 'autonomic instability... deconditioning, hypovolaemia or immune-or virus-mediated neuropathy,' while a 2022 paper by Chadda et al. posits that POTS is a common development as part of Long Covid, further suggesting that possible underlying mechanisms may include '...hypovolaemia, neurotropism, inflammation

---

57. Dani et al., 'Autonomic dysfunction in "long COVID": rationale, physiology and management strategies', 2021.

and autoimmunity.'[58] Therefore, it would seem that 'Long Covid', while the condition might have certain unique pathological mechanisms, is really just another name for ME/CFS and similar illnesses.

Given that great likelihood, it would seem more than feasible that the problem of hypovolemic thirst has skyrocketed in the last few years and, in actual fact, two recent research papers into the kinds of symptoms that occur in Long Covid would appear to support this possibility. In one paper (Davis et al., 'Characterizing long Covid in an international cohort: 7 months of symptoms and their impact', 2021), 3762 Long Covid patients answered surveys regarding their key symptoms. 35% of respondents cited 'extreme thirst' as a symptom. Meanwhile in an even larger study with a similar aim (Thaweethai et al., 'Development of a Definition of Post-acute Sequelae of SARS-CoV-2 Infection', 2023), 40% of the 9764 patients cited thirst as one of their main symptoms, leading the researchers to suggest that it should be considered as one of the 12 key symptoms that define Long Covid. The possible nature of this thirst is not explored in either paper but, from my perspective, I would imagine that it is driven by hypovolemia, at least for the most part.

***

So far in this chapter, I have put forward a basic model of how hypovolemic dehydration can explain a vicious cycle of excessive water intake and dilute urine along with hyponatraemia. I then proceeded to suggest that ME/CFS, POTS and Long Covid are illnesses in which, due to endogenous hypovolemia, patients could arguably suffer from hypovolemic thirst. We also explored the downregulation of the RAA axis and resultant low plasma volume as well as the diminished red blood cell volume, both factors which drive the hypovolemia within these illnesses. From all of

58.   Chadda et al., 'Long COVID-19 and Postural Orthostatic Tachycardia Syndrome - Is Dysautonomia to Be Blamed?', 2022.

these aspects, we have a plausible model for what is likely really going on in so-called 'Primary Polydipsia'.

If this model is correct, however, we should expect to see hints of it in the research published to date on psychogenic water drinking. By this I mean that, even though that research has never explicitly considered the possibility of a thirst caused by low blood volume, it may nevertheless have unwittingly stumbled upon findings that support such an hypothesis, even if the logical conclusion of those findings was not then followed. And, indeed, in reading through the research on 'Primary Polydipsia', I did find several papers that unknowingly supported my own hypothesis. This 'support' essentially adds weight to the idea that low blood volume has always been the real issue at play and so let us now turn to consider that research in more detail.

Clues Pointing to Hypovolemic Thirst in the Pre-Existing 'Primary Polydipsia' Literature

From the pre-existing literature, there are two papers in particular which inadvertently add major support to my hypothesis.

The first paper comes from Japan and was by Saruta et al. in 1982. Titled 'Evaluation of the renin-angiotensin system in diabetes insipidus and psychogenic polydipsia', the study involved administration of an angiotensin II analog in order to evaluate RAA axis activity, particularly in the form of renin activity, in patients with Diabetes Insipidus and with so-called Psychogenic Polydipsia. Such a study is ideal from the point of view of this book's hypothesis as it tests RAA axis function. Under normal circumstances, RAA axis activity should increase in response to angiotensin II administration. This is indeed what happened in the Diabetes Insipidus patients: all patients had a marked increase in renin activity, indicating a physiologically normal response. However, in all the so-called Primary Polydiptics, renin activity did not increase markedly at all: it remained low or normal. This is a clear indication of a blunted

RAA axis response. For the authors of the paper, this finding suggested that testing RAA axis activity could be useful for diagnostic procedures. This never became an established protocol, however, and uncovering the likely real significance of the differing RAA axes responses was not pursued by the authors. It is something however that entirely conforms with the hypothesis I am putting forward, namely that, in hypovolemic dehydration, the RAA axis is incapable of increasing its activity as it should. Was this study really just testing the RAA-axis of thirsty ME/CFS patients?

The second paper is particularly interesting. In my theoretical model of hypovolemic dehydration near the start of this chapter, I suggested that the endogenous solute loss will not only create a hypovolemic state but will also contribute to the development of hyponatraemia. If this is the case, it contradicts current teaching on Primary Polydipsia completely. Indeed, it is currently an *idée fixe* that the hyponatraemia results solely from the enormous quantities of ingested fluid and the inability of the kidneys to excrete that fluid in time. Under this view, the hyponatraemia is therefore purely the result of excessive water intake and the blame for it can be attributed solely to the patients' supposedly misplaced habits. In contrast, if it can be shown that the hyponatraemia is not only dilutional but that it also results from specific pathological mechanisms, then this would clearly imply that something organic is going on. This is what the second paper essentially points to. Written in 2003 by Musch et al. with the title 'Solute loss plays a major role in polydipsia-related hyponatraemia of both water drinkers and beer drinkers', the paper identified key evidence that the low blood sodium did not stem from the acute dilutional state alone but that the bodies of so-called Primary Polydiptics were also losing solute for some other reason. But how was this conclusion reached?

The striking abnormality observed in this paper was that the patients had a normal plasma protein concentration despite their hyponatraemic state. In the case of pure dilutional hyponatraemia, one would expect plasma protein concentration to lower as the result of an expanded extracellular space. In other words, the overall dilutional state should also dilute the plasma protein, thereby lowering its concentration. The fact that this did not happen indicates that there was more than just dilutional hyponatraemia at play and that the hyponatraemia must have also resulted from some other additional factor that created a significant solute loss. Indeed, from their analysis, Musch et al. suggested that the hyponatraemia likely stemmed 50% from solute loss and 50% from the dilutional state. However, the authors were unsure as to the reasons for this solute loss, writing:

> 'It is difficult to judge the cause of the solute deficit in polydip-sia-related hyponatremia...Defence mechanisms against extracel-lular fluid expansion, including inhibition of the renin-angioten-sin-aldosterone system and stimulation of natriuretic peptides, could be involved in solute loss of such patients.'

It is interesting that Musch posits an idea rather in line with this book's hypothesis, albeit from the standpoint of more standard textbook physiology (i.e. that the RAA axis may be downregulated to protect against fluid expansion rather than blunted as a matter of course as it is in ME/CFS). However, looking at this paper in the light of ME/CFS can completely render explicable the central mystery of the solute loss which it observed. For could it not be the case that the chronic suppression of the RAA-axis activity is the 'missing link' that was, in fact, the factor responsible for the solute-loss that was found in this study? I would suggest so. In this way, we have a strong indication that the hyponatrae-mia observed in so-called Primary Polydipsia patients is driven by the organic pathology of RAA axis suppression and not by a mentally ill habit.

From both of these papers, we therefore have a clear indication that there exist in so-called Primary Polydipsia strikingly different mechanisms from those which are most typically assumed. In the standard view, the condition hinges entirely on vasopressin-related functions and it is assumed that the hyponatraemia results purely from the amount of ingested fluid, both *idées fixes* that stem from regarding the condition purely through the lens of osmotic thirst. In contrast, the above papers suggest that vasopressin-related functions are not the real issue but that the initial key pathophysiological mechanism is more likely to be RAA axis suppression. Similarly, Musch's paper shows us that the high ingestion of fluid alone is unlikely to be the sole cause of the hyponatraemia, as is commonly assumed, but that the low blood sodium may also be driven by RAA axis downregulation. The findings from both of the above papers clearly contradict the general assumptions on which so-called Primary Polydipsia depends but, despite this, neither of these papers sparked further research nor did they lead to any challenges of the standard view of Primary Polydipsia.

Further Clues

In addition to the aforementioned two papers, there are other hints in the previous literature on Primary Polydipsia which can support the claims I make in this book, albeit to a lesser extent. In this case, one paper describes a case study in which a patient receiving a volume-boosting medication had a resolution of her symptoms, while there are also a couple of papers that support a possible link between so-called Primary Polydipsia and Myalgic Encephalomyelitis. All of these papers refer to specific and singular case studies and, therefore, the strength of their evidence is weaker. They are, nevertheless, worth discussing.

The first case report (Mellinger, 'Primary polydipsia. Syndrome of inappropriate thirst', 1983) describes a patient with 'lifelong severe polyuria and polydipsia'. Mellinger is quite clear that he believed his patient's suffering was real: 'This syndrome is not psychogenic polydipsia and it is not related to an emotional disturbance in any manner. During the years she was seeking medical help, the suggestion that these symptoms might represent a mental disorder added to the patient's distress.' Key for this observation was that the patient's polydipsia symptoms resolved when on Desmopressin, a synthetic form of vasopressin: after 0.1mg vasopressin every 12 hours, her crippling thirst went away and she drank a normal amount of fluid. Indeed, prior to the Desmopressin her daily fluid intake was 4.7 litres and her output was 4.3 litres. After Desmopressin, this dropped to an intake of 2.5 litres and an output of just 875ml.

For Mellinger, his patient was likely suffering from inappropriate thirst signals. Indeed, he suggested that her 'thirst stimulus was not inhibited by normal plasma osmolality' or, in other words, that there was a kind of inappropriate 'thirst reset' at play. However, the paper's data can also be read as supportive of my general hypothesis. Note the difference between the patient's fluid input (2.5 litres) and urine output (0.875ml) while on Desmopressin: 1.625 litres. While some of this water will have been lost through sweat, respiration and so forth, the remaining amount of fluid is very significant and would undoubtedly have boosted the patient's blood volume as a result. Is this the real reason why the patient reported relief? We cannot know nor can we rule out Mellinger's observations but it is a point that is worth considering. It is also notable that the patient reported that her prior symptoms tended to improve when she was pregnant. It is commonly observed that pregnant ME patients tend to experience a significant amelioration within their condition while carrying their child.[59] This is likely because pregnancy forcibly increases blood volume: indeed, plasma volume typically increases by 18%-29% in the 2nd trimester and by 42% in the third.[60] The

---

59. Schaterlee et al., 'A comparison of pregnancies that occur before and after the onset of chronic fatigue syndrome', 2004.

60. Aguree and Gernand, 'Plasma volume expansion across healthy pregnancy: a systematic review and meta-analysis of longitudinal studies', 2019.

fact that the patient in Mellinger's study had less thirst while pregnant would therefore be something in accordance with my general theory.

Another two case reports, both from India, support the possible link between so-called Primary Polydipsia and ME/CFS. The first (Bhatia et al., 'Psychogenic Polydipsia – Management Challenges', 2017) concerns the case study of a 35 year old man whose daily water intake had been around 10 litres for several years. While his medical team identified no organic cause and therefore diagnosed the patient as having psychogenic polydipsia, they missed one very important factor (italics my own):

> 'On elicitation of history from the patient, his wife and his brother who accompanied him, it was reported that the patient was apparently functioning well until 2 to 3 years ago *when he had an episode of fever following which he started reporting complaints of weakness and anxiety...* He reported that he would feel anxious and irritable if he was unable to get water or if family would stop him from taking water. His appetite had decreased and he had suffered loss of weight over the period of 2 years and had thoughts preoccupied with water intake. He would always keep a 2 litre bottle of water with him. He also lost interest in work and stopped going to work, *citing weakness and fatigability all through the day as the reason for absenteeism from work.*'

Clearly, this patient's history ties in precisely with the classic development pattern of ME/CFS: a viral trigger leading then to regular episodes of post-exertional malaise. From such a basis, it is perfectly feasible that the real reason for his thirst was hypovolemic dehydration as part of his condition. Knowledge about ME/CFS is almost non-existent among the vast majority of doctors, however, and, in this case, the likely real significance of the patient's medical history seems to have been lost.

The final case report is particularly interesting (Subramanian et al., 'Converging Neurobiological Evidence in Primary Polydipsia Resembling Obsessive Compulsive Disorder', 2017). The patient in this case, a 27 year old woman with no previous medical or psychiatric history, was admitted to emergency medical services after being rescued from an attempted suicide by hanging. The result of the suicide attempt had left her in a coma and brain scans revealed that she had an hypoxic brain injury. Her time in intensive care was traumatic. She developed ventilator-associated pneumonia followed by a delirium which lasted for two weeks. However, a brain MRI showed no structural abnormalities at that point.

In the six months following discharge, the patient developed new symptoms: poor concentration, stuttered speech, impulsivity, emotional lability, an unstable gait and memory impairment. She also started to drink enormous amounts of water: 12-14 litres per day. It was as part of the diagnostic process for this new symptom that the patient was ultimately given a diagnosis of Primary Polydipsia.

As part of these diagnostic procedures, the brain of the patient was scanned again, revealing a 'global hypometabolism due to ischemic injury especially in the basal ganglia and the cerebellum'. The hypometabolic state in the basal ganglia in particular suggested a causal link with OCD, as a hypometabolic basal ganglia has been implicated in that condition. From this basis, Subramanian posits that Primary Polydipsia may be 'neurobiologically related to OCD', therefore seemingly representing some kind of psychological 'compulsion' to drink a lot of water. However, this statement is rather at odds with the fact that this patient did not actually report any symptoms of OCD. As Subramanian also notes: 'No obsessions or compulsions were elicited in the Yale-Brown Obsessive-Compulsive Disorders Scale (Y-BOCS) checklist.' Subramanian admits that this last factor would normally make an OCD diagnosis unlikely in most cases but also suggests that, regarding this patient, the organic brain injury might result in a lack of patient awareness of their compulsive behaviours. He writes: 'A patient's report of intrusiveness, ego-dystonicity, and resistive attempts hold the key to diagnosing OCD as per classificatory systems in psychiatry. Nonreporting of such factors by our patient could be explained by an illness indifference commonly seen in OCD patients with an organic etiology – the hypoxic brain injury in our patient.'

While this might be the case, there are other ways of reading Subramanian's paper. In particular, we know that brain scans of ME/CFS patients have had similar findings. Indeed, a systematic review of 63 relevant papers, found that ME/CFS is associated with 'regional hypometabolism' of the brain.[61] Even more interestingly, hypometabolism of the basal ganglia has been particularly implicated in ME/CFS. In his 2014 paper ('Decreased Basal Ganglia Activation in Subjects with Chronic Fatigue Syndrome: Association with Symptoms of Fatigue'), Miller et al. found that ME/CFS is strongly associated with lowered functioning within the basal ganglia. That paper's abstract reads:

> 'Patients with chronic fatigue syndrome (CFS) have been shown to exhibit symptoms suggestive of decreased basal ganglia function including psychomotor slowing, which in turn was correlated with fatigue.... In order to directly test the hypothesis of decreased basal ganglia function in CFS, we used functional magnetic resonance imaging to examine neural activation in the basal ganglia to reward-processing (monetary gambling) ... Compared to non-fatigued controls, patients with CFS exhibited significantly decreased activation in the right caudate and right globus pallidus..... These data suggest that symptoms of fatigue in CFS subjects were associated with reduced responsivity of the basal ganglia, possibly involving the disruption of projections from the globus pallidus to thalamic and cortical networks.'

While we cannot know for sure what was going on with the patient in Subramanian's case report, it is feasible that she actually developed ME/CFS following the traumatic events she suffered (both the failed

---

61. Shan et al., 'Neuroimaging characteristics of myalgic encephalomyelitis/chronic fatigue syndrome (ME/CFS): a systematic review', 2020

hanging and its aftermath but also her physiologically devastating stay in intensive care). This is because ME/CFS can not only be triggered by viral illnesses but can also result from any other kind of trauma, broadly understood. When we consider that hypometabolism within the basal ganglia is a central characteristic of ME/CFS and that this patient suffered from that same hypometabolism, it is feasible that her extreme thirst might have actually stemmed from the development of ME/CFS and its characteristic hypovolemia. It is also noticeable that her baseline cortisol was below the reference range at 6.67 (normal range: 7-28), something which is highly suggestive of the hypocortical state that has been found in most studies that have examined cortisol in ME/CFS.[62] When we particularly reflect on the fact that the patient reported no actual OCD compulsions or obsessions, it seems even more likely that her basal ganglia abnormalities may really have resulted from the development of ME/CFS. In addition, decreased basal ganglia function in ME/CFS, as Miller notes, is also associated with 'psychomotor slowing' which may explain some of the other symptoms (such as the stuttered speech and unstable gait) that the patient developed. Obviously, Subramanian's perspective cannot be ruled out but, when we review this case study in light of ME/CFS research, it does seem more than possible that the patient might really have had ME/CFS and suffered from excessive thirst for that reason.

Conclusion

In this chapter, we have considered how the concept of hypovolemic dehydration can explain the same general symptom presentation that is observed in so-called 'Primary Polydipsia', that of unquenchable thirst, dilute urine and hyponatraemia. We then discussed in more detail the examples of ME/CFS, POTS and Long Covid and the hypovolemia that

---

62. Torres-Harding et al., 'The associations between basal salivary cortisol and illness symptomatology in chronic fatigue syndrome', 2008.

can be a central part of those illnesses, thereby providing us with a patient group that might suffer from endogenous hypovolemic thirst. We have also explored examples in the medical literature where previous Primary Polydipsia researchers may have unknowingly stumbled upon findings actually suggestive of hypovolemic dehydration. All in all, the discussion in this chapter has added many factors to the argument that hypovolemic thirst is what has likely always really been at play in so-called Primary Polydipsia.

But my hypothesis would mean rather little if patients with hypovolemic-illnesses, such as ME/CFS, were not also chronically thirsty. Indeed, if my hypothesis is correct, then one would expect a significant number of patients with that illness to report this symptom. And so now let us turn to consider evidence of this symptom among ME/CFS patients themselves and in their own words.

As we shall see, that evidence is quite overwhelming.

Chapter Three

Excessive Thirst in ME/CFS - The Examples of Patients

From our discussion so far, we can conclude that if there is one patient population that is likely to suffer from a previously unappreciated kind of polydipsia, namely one driven by low blood volume, it is those who suffer from ME/CFS and closely related illnesses. In line with this, therefore, let us now turn to consider evidence of this symptom as described by the patients themselves. For if my hypothesis is correct, excessive thirst and urination should be symptoms that have been frequently noted by patients within the ME/CFS community.

But before turning to the voices of patients, let us first consider how this symptom has been described by several doctors who specialise in ME/CFS.

Firstly, this phenomenon is rather colourfully depicted by Dr. Jacob Teitelbaum in the following way: 'ME/CFS patients drink like fish and pee like racehorses!'[63] Dr. Teitelbaum suggests that this thirst is the result of lowered vasopressin production and proposes additional dietary salt as the most effective remedy.[64]

---

63. Johnson C., 'Enhancing Blood Volume in Chronic Fatigue Syndrome (ME/CFS) and Fibromyalgia', Website: www.healthrising.org/treating-chronic-fatigue-syndrome/enhancing-blood-volume-in-chronic-fatigue-syndrome-mecfs-and-fibromyalgia/

64. *Ibid.*

Dr. David Bell, meanwhile, a now-retired physician who specialised in ME/CFS patients, had a particular interest in this problem. In a public lecture on hypovolemia in the illness, Dr. Bell noted that he had observed increased thirst in many of his patients who could drink 'up to three gallons' (11.5 litres) daily. Dr. Bell does not go so far as to suggest what might be driving this high intake of fluid but, interestingly, he does note that an endocrine colleague simply assumed that it must be Primary Polydipsia. The relevant extract from Dr. Bell's lecture reads as follows:

'There are several mechanisms that come into play when the blood volume falls. The first is the hormone ADH (anti-diuretic hormone) which is missing in diabetes insipidus (not sugar diabetes or diabetes mellitus). In diabetes insipidus an injury or tumor of the pituitary causes ADH production to halt and persons with this condition urinate a great deal and carry around water jugs with ice water (sound familiar?)

There have been a number of studies on DI and ADH and without going into details, ADH can be produced in persons with ME hypovolemia. It is just that the pituitary does not seem to think that the hypovolemia is wrong or bad, no big deal. However, something recognizes it as a big deal because people with ME can drink up to three gallons of water daily. When I asked an endocrinologist about this, he said it was "psychogenic water drinking."'[65]

From these two examples, we can see an awareness among ME/CFS physicians and researchers that polydipsia is a common feature of the illness. More precise mechanisms for this symptom are not hypothesised, however. Dr. Teitelbaum's suggestion that it is simply the result of lowered vasopressin is not, I think, the whole picture, as we know that both salt and water retention hormones are downregulated

---

65. Johnson C., 'Dr. David Bell on Low Blood Volume in Chronic Fatigue Syndrome', Website:https://www.healthrising.org/forums/resources/dr-david-bell-on-low-blood-volume-in-chronic-fatigue-syndrome.234/

in the illness, suggesting the problem is one primarily of blood and not of water. Dr. Bell, meanwhile, does suggest that 'something recognizes it [i.e. the hypovolemia] as a big deal' but does not make any definitive conclusions as to what this might be. As is evident from our discussion so far, I think he is indeed right that 'something' recognises the hypovolemia as a 'big deal' but that that 'something' is, in fact, simply the hypovolemic thirst mechanism.

Let us now turn to consider further evidence of this symptom in ME/CFS through the words of patients. How do they describe excessive thirst and what form does it take? And what kinds of treatments have they followed to improve this symptom?

Excessive Thirst in ME/CFS: The Examples of Patients

In order to compile this evidence, I turned to one prominent ME/CFS support forum, www.phoenixrising.me. What quickly became apparent is that the amount of evidence regarding the existence of this symptom is considerable, demonstrating both its frequency and often its severity. I have not included every comment on every forum post regarding this symptom but I have decided to include more evidence rather than less so as to really drive the point home regarding how a central a feature the symptom of excessive thirst can be for ME/CFS patients. The symptom is also discussed at other patient forums (such as www.healthrising.org) as well as on the POTS support forum at the Dysautonomia Information Network (www.dinet.org) but that evidence is not included here. Some might suggest the kind of evidence presented in this chapter suffers from a lack of larger context. One cannot know the precise history of each patient nor the exact reasons for their thirst which, conceivably, could be caused by something other than their primary illness. However, the larger context is that all of these patients have ME/CFS and, within that fact, it is notable that the descriptions of their thirst are remarkably homogeneous. With that in mind, I believe that the forum posts presented here add considerable weight to the idea that a previously unappreciated kind of polydipsia exists in ME/CFS.

I have divided the evidence into three sections: posts that describe the general nature of thirst in ME/CFS; posts that describe treatments that have improved this symptom and posts that discuss the (mis) diagnosis of ME/CFS patients with psychogenic polydipsia. In general, these posts speak for themselves but I make some general observations prior to each section. I have also edited the posts in some cases to remove superfluous material (e.g. 'hope you have a nice day' and the like) and occasionally corrected spelling errors. The username precedes each comment and the relevant forum thread for each range of posts can be found in the footnotes. I occasionally add an explanatory note in parentheses (i.e. [.....]).

Section 1: General Posts about Thirst in ME/CFS

Note here how the thirst is often described as having a tendency towards producing large quantities of dilute urine along with lower sodium levels; how it can be constant for some patients but, for others, intermittent and often coinciding with post-exertional malaise; how some patients describe this as being their worst symptom and as a kind of living nightmare.

1. Emmarose47: I'm always thirsty... I can't seem to quench my thirst... Is this a thing with CFS?[66]

2. Rebeccare: It seems to be a thing with dysautonomia and POTS, which many people with ME/CFS also have. When I wake up in the mornings and my symptoms are the worst, I am so thirsty all the time (and I'm always running to the bathroom!).

3. Heapsreal: Very common in CFS/ME. Drink like fish and pee like a racehorse.

---

66. Posts 1-13 are from the thread 'Is thirst a thing for us?' (https://forums.phoenix-rising.me/threads/is-thirst-a-thing-for-us.83297/)

4. Deb74: I struggle with thirst and am constantly drinking water and then I spend a lot of time going to the toilet. It is driving me mad. My urine is always clear...

5. L'engle: I'm often very thirsty as well as having dry throat and mouth. If I drink too much it just goes through me but other times I can drink a lot without a problem.

6. Keepswimming: A search brought up this thread, as I have just realised what an abnormally large amount I drink, and wondered if I was alone... The incontinence clinic asked me to keep a record of how much I'm drinking to make sure I'm getting at least 2 litres a day. Yesterday I drank a total of 4.5 litres, not sure what they're going to make of that!! So, I guess I can add thirst to my list of symptoms!!!

7. Wolfgang Amadeus: Raging nocturnal thirst was one of the most disturbing symptoms I had in the early days after my Covid infection (which is what triggered my ME/CFS).

8. Zebra: This has been a part of my illness experience for as long as I can remember. Excessive thirst, leads to excessive consumption of water, which leads to excessive urination. Over the years I've had several urine tests rejected by laboratories because the sample was too dilute. Additionally, I've had several comprehensive metabolic panels reveal very slightly low sodium in the blood. No doctor I've seen (and I've seen A LOT), has ever shown any curiosity about these symptoms or these findings, including an endocrinologist!

9. Replenished: For me it's my main symptom. Thirst and frequent urination were how it all started for me, to the point where I was tested for Diabetes Insipidus (lack of vasopressin/anti-diuretic hormone) and my results were borderline...to this day since this whole thing started

I've not had a day where I've not felt utterly thirsty and dehydrated. No matter what concoction of electrolytes etc I drink. It's awful.

10. Jim777: I don't know if this helps or not but I drank so much water when I did a 24 hour urine test that they could not measure it! And yes since the onset of my problem over 25 years ago I drink a lot of water and I am more thirsty than I ever was before the onset of this illness.

11. Before_the_Dawm: I tend to drink a decent amount of water, but it sometimes makes me feel really sick. I also constantly have a thirst (and) …. I constantly need to urinate. I've been tested for diabetes by the GP many times over the years due to this….I tend to stop drinking liquids by 7pm but I'm up at least 3 times in the night needing to go. I've been like this for many years.

12. Nord Wolf: I'm always thirsty and dehydrate quickly. I tend to drink room temp water with the slightest amount of salt in it to prevent overloading the kidneys and thyroid with too much water. The minute amount of salt in the water helps them to process it. My healthcare team told me the thirst symptom is common in people with ME/CFS and POTS, of which I have both.

13. Mouse girl: Yes, always thirsty, sometimes more than other times. I remember reading about the illness about 30 years ago when I was in my early years of being sick and someone said that they always knew the other CFS patients in a waiting room, because they always had huge water bottles they were drinking.

14. Seadragon: I suffer from extreme and constant thirst, excessive urination (at least every half an hour) and dehydrate very rapidly. No diabetes (of either type) and electrolytes (and everything else) all normal

on bloodwork and urine sample. Nothing shows up ever and my doctor shrugs her shoulders.[67]

15. gu3vara: I'm worried, I had those symptoms of dehydration for a while and it was getting better. But it's worse than ever now, feels like water goes straight through me, leaving me feeling dehydrated all over, skin, muscle, constipation, excessive thirst, dry mucus in nostrils, burning tears...and the worst, I'm twitching awfully, all over. My muscles are out of order when trying to walk.

16. Ocean: I'm not sure but I think dysautonomia can also affect some of this stuff too. I have an unusually high urine volume and often am the same way, just very dehydrated despite drinking a lot.

17. taniaaust1: I get that sometimes too... actually have it today. My skin is showing signs of dehydration (if I press on my finger, today its staying indented and I'm very thirsty). I've had days where I've drank 7 Litres of water in one day (I actually drank till I started throwing up water) and still been thirsty...some days my body just isn't holding its fluids. (I used to have this problem constantly but now it's just on some days). One of my sodium tests was low... I assume cause I didn't salt load enough that day for the fluid I drank. (I have POTS and I think my issue is part of all that).[68]

18. Bleusky: I'm posting on behalf of a friend who was diagnosed with ME a few years ago. She recovered and went into remission for a period, back to life, work etc. Unfortunately, a UTI infection (possibly) about a year ago set her back to a 24/7 bedbound state. In addition to fatigue,

---

67. Post 14 is from the thread 'Anything that can help with excessive thirst and urination and rapid dehydration?' (https://forums.phoenixrising.me/threads/anything-that-can-help-with-excessive-thirst-and-urination-and-rapid-dehydration.15053/).

68. Posts 15-17 are from the thread 'I feel very dehydrated no matter how much I drink' (https://forums.phoenixrising.me/showthread.php?16722-I-feel-very-dehy-drated-no-matter-how-much-I-drink)

her main symptoms are an abnormal thirst, lack of appetite, yellowish tongue, inflamed bladder, disturbed sleep due to frequent nocturnal urination. I wondered whether anybody has had to deal with this kind of symptom picture. In particular, an abnormal thirst and need to drink. Appetite is lacking and she can eat very little once a day, usually at night and only after drinking 6-7 pints of water which seems to stimulate a little appetite for food. Diabetes, including diabetes insipidus, have been ruled out by the doctors, so has any bladder infection that would explain discomfort in the pelvic area and frequent urination.

19. Sparrow: I don't know about the bladder issues, but I am chronically thirsty. That part seems to be common with ME. I'm especially thirsty when I'm overdoing it with activity.[69]

20. PatJ: I never drink just water because most of it goes *through* me instead of *into* me. Electrolyte drinks allow my body to hold onto water better than when using just water, but I still urinate very frequently. I have to find a balance point because after I pass a certain threshold my body increases urination to compensate for the excess fluids.[70]

21. Paul80: I've had this for a while. I need to drink a lot of water or I get dehydrated and I am constantly urinating. Even if I don't drink a lot I still need to urinate often. My doctor surgery has been really unhelpful in the past with my M.E. They have done blood tests in the past for the dehydration and they came back fine.[71]

---

69. Posts 18-19 are from the thread 'Abnormal thirst and chronic bladder issues' (https://forums.phoenixrising.me/threads/abnormal-thirst-and-chronic-bladder-issues.22230/)

70. Post 20 is from the thread 'dehydration' (https://forums.phoenixrising.me/threads/dehydration.50505/)

71. Post 21 is from 'Dehydration and frequent urination' (https://forums.phoenix-rising.me/threads/dehydration-and-frequent-urination.34433/)

22. Murph: You sound a *lot* like me! I eat insane amounts of salt. I drink maybe 10L of water a day and pee about the same! If I don't drink I feel terrible. I assume blood volume gets too low.[72]

23. Gingergrrl: ...the last few months I'm having an issue where I literally have to pee all night long. It wakes me up all throughout the night and is affecting my sleep and I feel more tired during the day. Sometimes I have to pee 2-3x per hour vs. other times I can go 1-2 hours in between having to pee.[73]

24. Replenished: I don't know what to do, I can't carry on living like this but nobody has any answers. The main issue I have is constant dry mouth and feeling completely depleted and dehydrated. That leads on to me feeling very weak and unwell. My urine is nearly always clear even if I drink very little. I am unable to retain fluids adequately. I have been tested for diabetes insipidus and the results came back as borderline. I do not concentrate urine as normal but it does not look like typical diabetes insipidus...I feel as though my life is slipping away from me.

25. Themjay: I have exactly the same issues and it was the first symptom I got investigated by the NHS nearly 20 years ago. I tried Desmopressin which just made me feel "wrong". I need to go to the toilet an average of 10 times a night - full bladder, clear urine just as you say. Sometimes only 10 minutes passes before the urge again. The other week I reached a new record of 17 visits between 1am & 8am. The doctors are

---

72. Post 22 is from the thread 'What causes dehydration/electrolyte imbalance' (https://forums.phoenixrising.me/threads/what-causes-dehydration-electrolyte-imbalance.77204/)

73. Post 23 is from the thread 'M.E./POTS – Treatment, medications, protocols to increase fluid retention, hydration and blood volume' (https://forums.phoenixrising.me/threads/m-e-pots-treatments-medications-protocols-to-increase-fluid-retention-hydration-and-blood-volume.89044/).

useless and it increases their suspicion that we are all anxiety-ridden hypochondriacs.[74]

26. CFS Warrior: I've been feeling super thirsty for several months now without the ability to feel hydrated. I drink at least 2 gallons of water a day. My skin is very dry even with lotion, which is unusual because I normally have oily skin. I have recently added extra salt to my meals as an experiment which has seemed to have helped some. I am unsure what is causing this and my doctor is unsure too. I have POTS which might have nothing or something to do with it. I know my medication is not causing this problem nor is consuming too much coffee or tea. The weather is not causing this either. I feel stuck.[75]

27. MeSci: At my worst I have had to endure having to urinate every 5-10 minutes for up to 4 hours, but mercifully it doesn't happen very often, as that is hellish, especially as it usually happens at night. On good days (also quite rare) my output is almost normal with little or no Desmopressin. Must be due to the fluctuations in ME.

28. Sidereal: I've never found an endocrinologist who was willing to help me with this problem, though even if I did, I think I would be too afraid to take Desmopressin. This drug is no joke; you can get water poisoning and die. Unlike some people on this thread with clear-cut DI [Diabetes Insipidus], like many others with ME, my DI is intermittent and seems to coincide with episodes of crashing, PEM [Post Exertional Malaise], monthly cycle or just a random flare in inflammation that I can't attribute to anything in particular. I will suddenly start dumping

---

74. Posts 24-25 are from the thread 'I cannot deal with this anymore – dry, depleted, dehydrated, weak, lifeless' (https://forums.phoenixrising.me/threads/i-cannot-deal-with-this-anymore-dry-depleted-dehydrated-weak-lifeless.82729/)

75. Post 26 is from the thread 'Feeling dehydrated despite large consumption of water' (https://forums.phoenixrising.me/blog-articles/feeling-dehydrated-de-spite-large-consumption-of-water.2365/)

enormous amounts of urine and electrolytes (judging by the volume and colour I would say it's both water and solute diuresis) and develop muscle weakness and fasciculations (well, worse than usual!) which I am able to counter somewhat by drinking more + constant sodium and potassium supplementation. This erratic nature of the problem makes me think I would be unable to dose this drug safely. This is probably my most frightening symptom.[76]

Section 2: Posts About Helpful Treatments for Excessive Thirst in ME/CFS

If we can ascertain the kinds of treatments that help ME/CFS patients with their excessive thirst, then we also have further indications as to the nature of the problem. Note in the following posts how many people improved this symptom by taking measures to increase blood volume (e.g. through increased dietary salt, the use of Flurinef, drinking Oral Rehydration Solution or having a saline IV). The question of possible treatments will be explored in more detail in the next chapter but for now it is worth noting that the following examples generally tend to suggest that thirst in ME/CFS stems from hypovolemia. In the main, efforts to boost plasma volume are discussed but a couple of patients found that their thirst improved from taking B12, something which has a role in increasing red blood cell production. Interestingly, there are a few other examples of treatments that successfully quenched the thirst (Low Dose Naltrexone in one case and coconut water in another, something which is high in potassium and not sodium) which may point to other additional aspects of the kind of thirst ME/CFS patients can experience. The final post in this section is of particular interest. It is the patient's record of a conversation with his doctor about this symptom. In this case, the doctor recommends that his dysautonomia patients only drink

---

76. Posts 27-28 are from 'Desmopressin (ADH) for polyuria (excessive urination)' (https://forums.phoenixrising.me/threads/Desmopressin-adh-for-polyuria-exces-sive-urination.32246/)

Oral Rehydration Solution as any plain water will just pull more sodium out of the body.

29. BrightCandle: For me the solution was electrolytes, I needed to take them in daily and I need a substantial amount of Magnesium per day, 1.5x the dose on the packet and that is alongside the electrolyte tablets I take with water and alongside a diet that includes a lot more natural magnesium. Doing this for months, the thirst problem gradually went away.[77]

30. Ema: Low aldosterone can make you dehydrated on a cellular level. It made me feel like my brain was shaking inside my head along with profound weakness/dizziness. If proper aldosterone testing (testing first thing AM after salt fasting for 24 hours) shows a deficiency, Florinef and increased salt consumption can solve the dehydration and increased urinary output symptoms in a hurry.[78]

31. LaurelW: I have had this problem [excessive thirst] in the past when I ate a very low-salt diet, and it went away when I raised my salt intake.[79]

32. Vincent: So over the last 3 years I've been to urgent care and the ER 5 times, the most recent 2 were last week. I'm permanently thirsty. I can only drink gatorade and I drink in excess of 25 8oz glasses per day, chugging it as fast as I can. My lips are always chapped and I get confused, feel sleepy when standing up, nauseous, and blurred vision. Everything but the nausea will mostly go away if I lay down. I have a

---

77. Post 29 is from the thread 'Is thirst a thing for us?' (https://forums.phoenixrising. me/threads/is-thirst-a-thing-for-us.83297/)

78. Post 30 is from the thread 'I feel very dehydrated no matter how much I drink', (https://forums.phoenixrising.me/showthread.php?16722-I-feel-very-dehydrated-no-matter-how-much-I-drink)

79. Post 31 is from the thread 'Abnormal thirst and chronic bladder issues' (https://forums.phoenixrising.me/threads/abnormal-thirst-and-chronic-bladder-issues.22230/)

feeling of derealization, trouble finding words, and trouble spelling. All I want to do is lay down all day. Now here is the thing, when I go to urgent care of the ER within minutes of them starting a saline drip I immediately feel better, like my brain is finally awake. As a teenager I did have orthostatic hypotension but now I do not; I acquired this after getting mono in 1993. I watched Dr. Rowe's presentation and I believe I might have low blood volume.[80]

33. **Seven7:** What nobody ever told me was that sometimes you need more than water. So I was dehydrated but I kept drinking water.... The more water I drank, the worse it got. Then I was told about the salt and potassium so I am doing salted pistachios as snack, and a 1/2 to 1 bottle of Pedialite a day (until lips are not dry) I can tell the difference in my heart rate variability, it becomes more stable. Don't get as dizzy...General malaise is better.

34. Sparrow: From the information I've gathered, I would very firmly say that it [excessive thirst] is a big issue for us. There is a lot of information out there to indicate that we have a lower volume of blood than the average healthy person, so we may be in legitimate need of more fluids to fill out what we do have. There is also some evidence to indicate that something may occasionally be off with our anti-diuretic hormone, so we would consequently lose more water from our body than others. Not sure if the two are connected, but both seem like likely connections to why we're so thirsty. And yes, I am crazy thirsty all the time. Beverages with electrolytes and about three litres or more of water per day have helped me some. I do notice that I seem to feel worse if I don't drink enough a couple of days in a row. And anything that dries me out normally (like coffee) is enough to push me into a pretty major slump now.

---

80. Post 32 is from the thread 'All the symptoms of dehydration, but electrolytes fine'(https://forums.phoenixrising.me/threads/all-the-symptoms-of-dehydration-but-electrolytes-are-fine.22138/)

35. Jstefi: I also have had this problem, and find that Gatorade helps a great deal. I go through a 2 liter bottle in about 4 days. I can't imagine life without it.[81]

36. Harmen: My fatigue is lifted immensely if I supplement huge amounts of salt (3~4 teaspoons if I am low). Constipation, out of breath, bonking slow beating heart, fatigue, cramps, extreme urination (like within 10 minutes after drinking it is peed out already), extreme thirst, no hunger etc all are relieved after 3 tsp of sea salt. Sleep is improved too.[82]

37. Replenished: I most certainly have POTS as well now. At the end of last week I got to the point where I was just so depleted, dehydrated and felt my blood/hydration volume was so low that I needed to do something and therefore decided to start taking some of the Fludrocortisone I had from a previous prescription to try and create some water retention. The Fludrocortisone does seem to have reduced my dehydration somewhat. I'm nowhere near normal/replenished/hydrated but I'm not absolutely unbearably dehydrated like I typically am and I'm urinating less.[83]

38. Manasi12: I have this similar problem, I can't retain water in my body. This is due to hypovolemia. It is really worse in morning. If I eat something salty and take water along with it, I feel better. Otherwise I'm on the verge of collapse. Fludrocortisone has improved this symptom.[84]

---

81. Posts 33-35 are from the thread 'Have you had dehydration?' (https://forums.phoenixrising.me/threads/have-you-had-dehydration.14339/)

82. Post 36 is from the thread 'Hyponatremia as a cause? Salt deficiency, dehydration, too much peeing' (https://forums.phoenixrising.me/threads/hyponatremia-as-a-cause-salt-deficiency-dehydration-too-much-peeing.7412/)

83. Post 37 from is from the thread 'Ongoing Dehydration – Best medication to use long term to intentionally increase water retention?' (https://forums.phoenixrising.me/threads/ongoing-dehydration-best-medication-to-use-long-term-to-intentionally-increase-water-retention.89002/)

84. Post 38 is from the thread 'I cannot deal with this anymore – Dry, depleted, dehydrated, weak, lifeless' (https://forums.phoenixrising.me/threads/i-cannot-deal-with-this-anymore-dry-depleted-dehydrated-weak-lifeless.82729/)

39. Allyson: Are polyuria, nocturia and polydipsia acknowledged symptoms of ME please? Many PWME [People with ME] whom I ask have them....For me, intramuscular B12 injections improve [this symptom] for a week or two – i.e. the polyuria stops - then returns after the injection wears off...IM B12 is something that helps a lot of people with ME - maybe this is why...apparently it is used to build connective tissue and also boosts blood volume.

40. Stridor: By July 2012, I was urinating over 20 times a day - with 4 and sometimes 5 times a night. I never did get an accurate count as I was too apathetic and fogged. After supper was the worst - I'd go 6+ times during a movie. There was an immediate marked improvement with mB12 [methylated B12] and the symptom was completely resolved within a week. I am up 0-1 times a night now which is OK for a guy my age.

41. Taniaaust1: Florinef has made a difference and I pee far less with it (about once a night, occasionally twice on the 2.5 pill dose I'm on currently). ...At one point I was having to drink so much that I was peeing twice an hour sometimes...I collapsed with dehydration last summer after drinking over 4L of fluid that day and the other day when I ended up collapsed and having to be ambulanced to hospital, I noticed after a couple of hours there, my lips were cracking due to dryness (the nurse also noticed and noted it in their report). My body just really struggles to hold onto its fluids.[85]

42. Mellster: LDN [low dose naltrexone] cut down my night-time urination and got it back to normal last year.

43. Meadow: I had the very same thing for many, many months. I was so thirsty that I drank so much water to the point of feeling water-

---

85. Posts 39-41 are from the thread 'Polyuria, nocturia and Polydipsia—ME symptoms?' (https://forums.phoenixrising.me/threads/polyuria-nocturia-and-poly-dipsia-me-symptoms.27568/)

logged, nauseated, etc, yet it never helped. I urinated excessively and I constantly felt dehydrated. I too did the 24 hour urine test - it was a cortisol related test if I recall properly - and if it had been 25 hours I think I would have needed another bottle – we are talking the size of a gas can. I tried making my own concoctions too after researching dehydration, but it did not really work. I had an opportunity to talk with an exceptional nutritionist and he recommended coconut water. He said that it is high in potassium and does not have all of the crap that sports drinks have in them. I buy the kinds without added sugar etc, just plain natural coconut water. I can tell you that it definitely quenched my thirst in ways that plain water could not. I still drink water regularly, but not gallons (so it seemed) hourly, and when the feeling comes on that I am getting thirsty/dehydrated and water is not cutting it, I go for the coconut water.[86]

44. GlassHouse:

Dr. Alan Pocinki has been researching this in his dysautonomia patients. Our conversation was like this:

Me: "I thought my tethered cord was getting worse because I have to pee at least every half hour. I got a urine hat to measure it because I was worried about retention but I'm peeing at least 300 mL each time, so my bladder is actually full when I feel like I have to pee. It's just full all the time and I pee at least 7 litres every day."

Him: "The next obvious question is where is all that fluid coming from?"

Me: "It's from what I drink. I tried to record that too and it seemed about equal. But I can't drink LESS because even drinking this much I feel like

---

86. Posts 42-43 are from the thread 'Anything that can help with excessive thirst and urination and rapid dehydration???' (https://forums.phoenixrising.me/threads/anything-that-can-help-with-excessive-thirst-and-urination-and-rapid-dehydration.15053/)

I'm dying of thirst! My mouth is dry, my skin is dry, surgeons have said all my tissues are dry."

Him: "You know, every single one of my patients tells me the same thing: 'I drink all the time but I'm always thirsty.' There seems to be something affecting dysautonomia patients' kidneys causing salt wasting. For some reason your bodies don't hold onto salt so you don't hold onto fluids."

Me: "I already drown all my food in salt. There's no way I could stand more."

Him: "You're probably not getting as much salt as you think. I've been measuring electrolytes in my patients' blood and am consistently finding you aren't getting enough salt, despite everyone trying to salt load. You need to drink electrolytes."

Me: "Oh I already do! I drink a ton of Vitalyte every day but I'm still super thirsty."

Him: "But are you also drinking plain water or tea or anything else?"

Me: "Well, yeah."

Him: "Unfortunately that's the problem. The water is washing out the electrolytes. It wouldn't be an issue for a healthy person, but for someone with dysautonomia the water counteracts the electrolyte drink."

Me: "So what do I do?"

Him: "You need to only drink salty electrolyte drinks, no plain water, all day."

Me: "That's impossible! The salt will make me more thirsty!"

Him: "You would think, but it's actually the opposite. Patients always think they'll feel more thirsty but it's the opposite."

So I tried it. I bought some LMNT pouches. I thought they tasted like drinking the ocean, and it was hard not to grab some water after but within 3 hours I got used to it (I also switched to cutting the LMNT with Vitalyte. It's more palatable). It was so weird, I peed a normal number of times and didn't have the urgency that came with my bladder filling all the way up within literally 20 min of drinking a few sips of water.

I still drink a cup of tea or decaf coffee but I'll try to only drink the salt drink. The salt drink has massively helped my thirst and urinary frequency/urgency. It's one of the few things that made a massive quality of life improvement for me. The only downside is that it's hard to adhere to the no other drinks rule. I like herbal tea, decaf coffee, and very occasionally a soda. Also, it doesn't taste great.[87]

Section Three: Posts about ME/CFS Patients Who Have Been Diagnosed with 'Primary Polydipsia'

In light of this book's thesis, one would expect to find some cases online where ME/CFS patients received a (mis)diagnosis of psychological over drinking of fluids. There were several such cases on the phoenixrising.me forum which are presented here.

45. MeSci: My own doctors were entirely useless when I went to them with excessive urine production (polyuria) and thirst. That includes the consultant. I did end up getting significant discomfort in the bladder, probably due to the muscles being exhausted by repeated filling and emptying. My thirst was due to the excessive fluid loss, but doctors persisted in claiming that it was the other way round - that my polyuria was due to 'primary polydipsia' - excessive fluid consumption. A few

---

87. Post 44 is from the thread 'Has anyone been diagnosed with Primary Polydipsia (compulsive water drinking)?' (https://forums.phoenixrising.me/threads/has-any-one-been-diagnosed-with-primary-polydipsia-compulsive-water-drinking.88343/)

internet searches will find medical claims that this is common in 'anxious middle-aged women.' Does this psychologization ring any bells...?[88]

46. Rachel Straub: I was diagnosed with psychogenic polydipsia by a world-renowned endocrinologist. I was drinking 2 gallons of water per day. I was also diagnosed with congenital neutropenia by a hematologist, which supposedly made me more susceptible to illness. I also had a 10+ year history of amenorrhea and was given female hormones for years. The doctors of endless specialities were ALL wrong... all these issues resolved once I was given thyroid medication (despite normal labs). Specifically, I required both Armour Thyroid and Levothyroxine. This all happened before I developed severe ME/CFS in 2013, which resulted in me becoming predominantly bedridden. You can read about this in my Case Report ('Chronic Fatigue Syndrome: A Case Report Highlighting Diagnosing and Treatment Challenges and the Possibility of Jarisch-Herxheimer Reactions if High Infectious Loads Are Present').[89] I was able to recover after 4.5 years of treatment (under the care of a MD, PhD) and return to grad school in 2017. However, I did relapse soon after resuming grad school (but that's another story). Nonetheless, I just finished my PhD at the University of Southern California, so there is hope. I am not 100% recovered, but I am improving.[90]

47. Pyrrhus: The sad thing is that some doctors see drinking too much liquid as a psychiatric condition called [psychological] "polydipsia". I know of one ME patient who was hospitalized and the doctors intention-

---

88. Post 45 is from the thread 'Abnormal thirst and chronic bladder issues' (https://forums.phoenixrising.me/threads/abnormal-thirst-and-chronic-bladder-issues.22230/)

89. Rachel Straub's case report is available at: https://pubmed.ncbi.nlm.nih.gov/34828583/

90. Post 46 is from the thread 'Has anyone been diagnosed with Primary Polydipsia (compulsive water drinking)?' (https://forums.phoenixrising.me/threads/has-any-one-been-diagnosed-with-primary-polydipsia-compulsive-water-drinking.88343/)

ally withheld water from the ME patient because they said the patient was suffering from psychological polydipsia.[91]

Conclusion

In this chapter, I have let ME/CFS patients tell their own story. In doing so, we have seen how the polydipsia symptoms can be constant, disruptive and, at times, severe. We have seen that the symptom presentation conforms with the typical one seen in so-called 'Primary Polydipsia', i.e. overly dilute urine along with low blood sodium levels and we have seen how efforts to boost blood volume tend to improve symptoms for patients. All of the evidence presented here therefore is in accordance with the general premise of this book.

We have just seen how measures to counteract hypovolemia have aided ME/CFS patients in practice. But how can we conceptualise, in a much broader way, treatment strategies for hypovolemic dehydration? In particular, how, in a hospital setting, should the more acute manifestations of hypovolemic thirst be treated? What should be the first priorities in treating patients with hypovolemic dehydration if they are also, say, profoundly hyponatraemic? What kind of messaging should doctors give such patients in order to get them 'on side'? How might you test for hypovolemic dehydration? And, once the acute phase has passed, what kind of lifestyle changes, supplements and medications might be employed on a daily basis to manage this condition?

Let us now turn to consider the question of treating hypovolemic dehydration in much more detail.

---

91. Post 47 from the thread 'Have to drink tons and tons of water or I'm dizzy' (https://forums.phoenixrising.me/threads/have-to-drink-tons-and-tons-of-water-or-im-dizzy.84931/)

Chapter Four

Treating Hypovolemic Dehydration

I f it is true that so-called compulsive water drinkers are actually suffering from a real physiological thirst as the result of a deficit of blood, then how should this symptom be treated? The answer, I believe, should depend on the current state of the patient and whether they are in an acute phase (i.e. drinking enormous quantities of water and likely hyponatraemic) or a stable phase (drinking under control with normal blood sodium levels). If the former, the first aim of treatment must be to restore normal blood sodium levels and the ability, at least to a significant degree, to produce concentrated urine. As I will explain shortly, it is likely that without these prerequisites, all attempts at assuaging the thirst of the patient will fail. If the patient is in a stable phase, treatment should be far more straightforward and relate largely to daily management, supplement and/or medication strategies, all of which I will discuss in this chapter. Having said that, if the concept of hypovolemic thirst is validated, then minds more scientific than my own would be far better placed to formulate treatment plans. The observations in this chapter are largely based on, and therefore necessarily limited by, my own personal experience and, at various points in the chapter, I will describe how I reached my primary recommendations based on my own experiments.

Treatment in the Acute Phase

It is essential to realise that, in the acute phase (for which treatment will most likely be in an hospital environment), the thirst experienced by a patient with hypovolemic dehydration is extreme: their whole body is racked with a thirst beyond the imagination of a healthy person. As such, the patient will go to considerable lengths to drink large quantities of water. This is one reason why so-called Primary Polydiptics can look 'mentally ill' from the outside: their entire behaviour is focussed on where they can get their next drink. The reason for this is simple. Thirst represents a basic survival need. In the same way that someone who is being suffocated can only think of how to get their next breath, someone who is suffering from extreme thirst is necessarily only focussed on quenching it. Given the physiological state of the patient, their behaviour makes perfect sense. The danger, of course, is that since the patient is applying the wrong remedy to their problem, they actually risk worsening their situation to the point of irreversible hyponatraemia-induced brain damage and perhaps even to the point of death.

Therefore, the kind of messaging given to such patients needs to get them 'on side' and thereby ensure their compliance. Clear and compassionate messaging such as the following could be imparted to the patient:

- Your thirst is actually not because of a lack of water but a lack of blood. Your body isn't able to maintain normal blood levels like a healthy person.

- The thirst you feel is very real but drinking more and more water can never fix it: you'll just pee it all out and your blood volume will remain low. Only concentrated fluids can increase your blood volume. You have been applying the wrong solution to the problem and that mistake is what has perpetuated your symptoms.

- We must resolve your hyponatraemic state as this is dangerous and a necessary precursor to successful treatment. You will therefore need to drink a limited amount of water, as defined by us, until this is resolved. You may even need to abstain from all fluids for a period so as to help your body 'reset', as best as is possible, its sodium levels and water & salt retention hormones.

- Your thirst will remain during this period. It may get worse or better at times but you need to tolerate it. After your blood sodium normalises and once we can apply appropriate treatments, I promise you that your thirst will improve. It will be nothing like what you are currently experiencing.

This kind of optimistic messaging should get the patient on board and willing to tolerate their current thirst level with a view to a treatment plan that will ameliorate their symptoms further down the road. These patients are not mentally ill and should respond to the concept and implications of hypovolemic dehydration with relief and co-operation. In contrast, the current messaging given to patients as a result of the 'Primary Polydipsia' model almost certainly guarantees non-compliance. Telling someone who is suffering from the worst thirst of their life that there is no physiological reason for them to be so thirsty must probably rank among the worst of all possible kinds of medical advice. It gives the patient no hope whatsoever. *I know I am stuck in a nightmare of extreme thirst but the doctor cannot help me and does not listen to what I say.* With no hope of successful treatment nor any sign that the doctor understands them, what will such patients do but continue to down enormous quantities of fluid? After all, that, it would reasonably seem to them, is precisely what their body is telling them to do. On the flip side, for the doctor overseeing their care, this behaviour only 'confirms' the supposed mental instability of the patient. *Why are they still drinking so much when I told them not to? There is no reason for them to drink so much water! They really must be mentally ill.* It is hard to imagine a greater mismatch between patient experience and medical textbook than this scenario.

With the patient on side, the most important aim then becomes the restoration of normal blood sodium levels and of the ability to produce concentrated urine. This is because the consistency of blood is supposed to be within certain physiological norms and a successful effort to expand plasma volume will depend on the presence of this normal consistency: there will then be a 'platform' which you can 'top up'. Similarly, the ability to produce some vasopressin, and therefore concentrated urine, is an important step towards maintaining blood's proper consistency. Due to the downregulation of the RAA and HPA axes, it may be that the vasopressin response will also be blunted. In fact, it almost certainly will be. A blunted response is still more useful than the complete vasopressin suppression that a high intake of water will have created, however. Some concentrated urine is better than urine that is ultra-dilute. Water and salt retention mechanisms are downregulated in hypovolemic dehydration but not obliterated completely (if this were the case, the patient would be dead). In other words, the relevant hormones are too low relative to the patient's true physiological needs with the result that a hypovolemic state has been created and subsequently maintained. It is important to find the patient's true baseline for water and salt retention so that the patient's body can then 'work with' the medical interventions chosen to expand blood volume.

Ideally, these aims could be achieved simply by restricting daily fluid intake (e.g. < 1.5 litres daily). However, it may be necessary, or even optimal in some cases, to cease fluid intake altogether. In this way, the current 'Water Deprivation Test' could be reconsidered as a treatment to 'reset' the body's sodium levels and kick, at least to some degree, vasopressin back into action. Of course, this is not an easy treatment for the patient to undergo: it is physically very demanding.

It may nevertheless be the most effective means to restart the relevant physiological mechanisms (as well as ruling out Diabetes Insipidus, if this is deemed necessary for the patient in question). In my own case, I believe the water deprivation test (in which I did not drink any fluids for 22 hours) was actually a key turning point in my condition. After around 18 hours, my blood sodium levels normalised and I started to produce concentrated urine. At the exact same moment, my thirst lessened by around 70%. I believe that this last point offers a crucial insight into the need for appropriately concentrated blood in the treatment of hypovolemic dehydration. It seems logical that the hypovolemic thirst centre will be much 'happier' once it detects that the blood is of a normal concentration again. It was certainly strange for someone accustomed to drinking huge quantities of fluid to find that 18 hours of drinking nothing at all actually lessened my thirst but this fact, if anything, adds further weight to the idea that the problem I faced was all to do with blood and not with water.

In my view, therefore, treatment in the more acute phase will depend on compassionate and clear messaging as to the nature of the problem so as to ensure patient compliance. Once that is achieved, the most important element then becomes undoing the damage of the high water intake, namely the almost total vasopressin-suppression and the low blood sodium. Once these have been corrected, as far as is possible, the patient's body will then be more receptive to treatments that can boost blood volume, thereby allowing them to assuage their thirst on an ongoing basis.

But how should one test for hypovolemic dehydration in a hospital setting? The water deprivation test could still be used, albeit with a result of concentrated urine not seen as indicating psychogenic water drinking but rather as pointing to the strong likelihood of hypovolemia-driven thirst. Of course, the water deprivation test is still helpful to rule out Diabetes Insipidus even if the juxtaposition of that condition alongside so-called Primary Polydipsia has always been misguided. Diabetes Insipidus is all about vasopressin while so-called Primary Polydipsia has, from a causal perspective, relatively little to do with that hormone. However, ultimately, it seems to me that, if hypovolemic thirst becomes a recognised condition, then new diagnostic procedures will need to be developed: perhaps there could be a safe way of testing RAA axis function with a view to detecting any suppression? Or maybe technology in this day and age could come up with even neater solutions. I recently came across a new machine that is in development, a blood volume analyser from Detalo Health (detalo-health.com), which might be ideal. That said, I have also read that some tools to measure blood volume might not be as sensitive as needed when it comes to ME/CFS patients. Perhaps ME/CFS researchers might be best placed to advise on the question of how to measure blood volume status quickly and efficiently in a hospital setting.

In any event, once the acute phase has passed, what kind of treatments could then be applied to help the patient manage their condition?

Daily Management of Hypovolemic Dehydration: The Role of Dietary Salt

One simple answer might involve increasing the amount of dietary salt and this would likely be a generally good idea for hypovolemic patients (indeed, many ME and POTS patients, so as to expand blood volume, are advised to 'salt load' to manage their condition).[92] This strategy will certainly increase plasma volume. For example, in a study on the effects of both high dietary salt (> 12 grams daily) and low dietary salt (< 3 grams daily) on Type I Diabetics, plasma volume increased from 3.2 to 3.5 litres on the high salt diet.[93] In that same study, cardiac output also increased

92. See Rowe P., 'General Information Brochure on Orthostatic Intolerance and its Treatment' (https://www.dysautonomiainternational.org/pdf/RoweOIsummary.pdf).

93. Wenstedt et al., 'Effect of high-salt diet on blood pressure and body fluid composition in patients with type 1 diabetes: randomized controlled intervention trial', 2020.

from 6.6 to 7.2 litres per minute. Such increases are clearly significant and could be very helpful in the context of hypovolemic dehydration.

The question, however, is whether the payoff of such a high salt diet is worth it. Indeed, such a high amount of salt is not benign, particularly because the body is not actually able to process safely such a high quantity of dietary salt. In the past it was thought that excessive dietary salt simply stayed temporarily in the bloodstream, increasing plasma volume and therefore blood pressure, before being excreted efficiently by the kidneys. Under this view, the supposed dangers of salt related only to its capacity to raise blood pressure by increasing extracellular fluid. Now, however, there is emerging evidence of a whole range of other negative effects of excessive dietary salt. While some ingested salt will of course boost blood volume, we now know that the rest is capable of leaving the bloodstream and damaging many other parts of the body. As a result, excessive salt can lead to: a damaged endothelium,[94] raised cortisol,[95] mitochondrial dysfunction,[96] gut dysbiosis,[97] excessive vasoconstriction along with reduced cerebral blood flow,[98] depression,[99] and, at amounts of 12 grams per day, muscle wasting[100] and many other

---

94. Edwards and Farquhar, 'Vascular Effects of Dietary Salt', 2015.

95. Baudrand et al., 'High sodium intake is associated with increased glucocorticoid production, insulin resistance and metabolic syndrome', 2014.

96. Geisberger et al., 'Salt Transiently Inhibits Mitochondrial Energetics in Mononuclear Phagocytes', 2021.

97. Ferguson et al., 'High dietary salt-induced DC activation underlies microbial dysbiosis-associated hypertension', 2019.

98. Faraco et al., 'Dietary salt promotes neurovascular and cognitive dysfunction through a gut-initiated TH17 response', 2018.

99. Mrug et al., 'Sodium and potassium excretion predict increased depression in urban adolescents', 2019.

100. Titze et al., 'Increased salt consumption induces body water conservation and decreases fluid intake', 2017.

things besides.[101] Indeed, excessive salt can actually permeate the blood vessel endothelium and become deposited in the skin.[102] In addition, the very nature of salt is, of course, dehydrating (in the conventional sense). There is a reason why drinking seawater can kill you. Once you ingest salt, it pulls water out of nearby cells via the process of osmosis, thereby dehydrating them. The body then must pull water back into the cells from extracellular fluid, but the process by which this happens is quite laborious and it takes time to repair the cellular damage that has been caused.[103] In this way, physiologically speaking, excessive salt represents a significant stressor for the body. Ideally, hypovolemic dehydration should not be treated in such a way that a whole host of new, negative side-effects are also created. That would simply be to solve one problem while creating another.

It is also helpful to look to nature and, in particular, to the examples of our forebears. Interestingly, traditional hunter-gatherer tribes do not consume significant amounts of salt. A 2015 paper[104] which reviewed the salt intake of contemporary hunter-gatherer tribes concluded that an ancestral level of salt consumption was probably no more than 2.5 grams daily. Among some tribes, however, salt intake was much lower even than that. The Yanomamo Indians of Brazil, for example, only have 0.1 grams of salt per day. Clearly, under healthy circumstances, the human body is capable of surviving, and thriving, on a very low intake of salt. This is consistent with the fact that, for most of their evolution, humans have had limited access to salt. Indeed, hunter-gatherer tribes, unless

---

101. For an overview of recent findings in salt-related research, see Robinson et al., 'The Influence of Dietary Salt Beyond Blood Pressure', 2019.

102. Selvarajah, 'Skin Sodium and Hypertension: A Paradigm Shift?', 2019.

103. Nunes et al., 'Ionic imbalance, in addition to molecular crowding, abates cytoskeletal dynamics and vesicle motility during hypertonic stress', 2015.

104. Campbell et al., 'Proposed Nomenclature for Salt Intake and for Reductions in Dietary Salt', 2015.

they lived close to the sea, would only really have had access to salt in the blood and meat of the animals they killed, otherwise consuming only trace amounts in their plant foods. Access to salt increased with the advent of salt mining but this arrived relatively late in human history with the dawn of more agricultural societies. The use of salt as a preservative made it highly attractive and it wormed its way into general human usage as a result. This makes excessive salt consumption a product of civilisation, therefore, and this is something which suggests that eating high amounts of it is neither natural nor necessarily a good idea.

On the other hand, patients with hypovolemic dehydration are not lithe hunter-gatherers and their bodies struggle to hold onto salt in a profound way due to illness. A daily diet of just 2.5 grams of dietary salt may do such patients no favours. A low salt diet could be very dangerous for some patients with hypovolemic dehydration (indeed, I believe this applied in my own case during the worst of my thirst-related episodes: I had religiously avoided salt, mistakenly believing that it would only increase my thirst!). The dose determines the poison. The important thing, in my opinion, is to understand that a high salt intake is not necessarily benign, contrary to what is claimed by some popular health influencers. In particular, given that Prof. Scheibenbogen, as we discussed in chapter two, has identified that both excessive vasoconstriction and vasodilation-impairment play a key role in ME/CFS, the capacity of salt to increase vasoconstriction might only worsen this problem and thereby place additional limits on the already global hypoperfusion that occurs within the illness. Indeed, a meal with just four grams of salt is capable of reducing postprandial vasodilation by 50%.[105]

All in all, I think hypovolemic patients should aim for a moderate amount of dietary salt, enough to help combat their hypovolemic thirst while also avoiding the deleterious effects of too much salt. In my own

105. Dickinson, 'Endothelial function is impaired after a high-salt meal in healthy subjects', 2019.

case, I find that around four to five grams of total dietary salt per day seems to achieve both those aims (indeed, such an amount of salt almost seems 'sweet' to my tastebuds), but each patient will have to work out what is most effective for them.

But this is far from being the whole story. Four or five grams of dietary salt will only have a modest impact on hypovolemic thirst and is merely a foundational strategy. What other kinds of more targeted options could be employed? Perhaps it would be interesting to consider next what nature itself would suggest. For the hypovolemic thirst mechanism was created by evolution and, as such, there is likely a natural 'solution' for it as well. What might that be?

Nature's Likely Solution to Hypovolemic Thirst

I would imagine that the natural remedy for hypovolemic thirst is a simple one. Indeed, when the body is thirsty because of a lack of water, the solution is to drink some water. Similarly, when the body is thirsty because of a lack of blood.....well, I hesitate to write it and my apologies for any squeamishness I may cause, but if the body is thirsty because of a lack of blood, nature's likely solution is probably for us to.....drink some blood. For what, in the natural world, could be better constituted to boost blood volume than blood itself?

It might be easy to dismiss this idea from our more modern and sanitized consciousness but if nature has gone so far as to create a hypovolemic thirst mechanism, then it makes equal sense that there must exist an evolutionarily appropriate means for assuaging that mechanism. If salt itself was not always readily available for hunter gatherer tribes, then the only other significant way to boost blood volume would have been to drink blood. Perhaps the Maasai tribes of Kenya and Tanzania who routinely blood let their cattle for a cup of blood are onto something.

So clearly all doctors should advise their patients with hypovolemic dehydration to pop down to the local butcher and put in an order for a daily pint of blood. There, problem solved! Well, perhaps not.... while a study examining the effect of daily blood consumption in this patient population would be fascinating, one imagines that patient buy-in might be lacking. The obvious fact is that, although this might be nature's natural solution, drinking blood today is culturally inappropriate and may be dangerously unhygienic. In essence, we live in an environment where nature's probable solution to this serious medical issue is simply not feasible.

If nature's likely natural solution is a no-go, then what further options remain? I believe that the answer to what is the safest and probably most effective treatment will actually still involve increasing one's salt intake but in a way which purely boosts blood volume and which does not otherwise cause the various harms of excessive dietary salt. But how can this be done? Luckily, there is a specific medical formulation that is able to achieve precisely this.

Oral Rehydration Solution to the Rescue: The Best Remedy for Hypovolemic Dehydration?

Oral Rehydration Solution (ORS) is a combination of salt, potassium and glucose prepared according to a specific formula devised by the World Health Organisation (WHO). ORS is particularly effective in combatting the significant fluid loss that occurs during diarrhoea. Indeed, for this purpose, ORS is a simple remedy that has saved countless lives (particularly in the developing world) and, in general, most people will probably be familiar with ORS from having taken it after a bout of vomiting or diarrhoea. In the UK, the most commonly available form of ORS is known as Dioralyte. In the US, various forms exist, including Pedialyte and Normalyte. The reason that ORS is so effective at counteracting fluid loss stems from the use of glucose in the solution. This is because our intestines are capable of almost completely transporting salt into the bloodstream as long as it is accompanied by a specific amount of glucose. This mechanism is called the 'salt-glucose co-transport carrier'.

While this is highly beneficial for the complications of excessive diarrhoea, ORS also represents an effective, if temporary, remedy for hypovolemia. A basic rule of physiology is that water follows salt. When you drink ORS, it is not just the case that additional salt will end up in your bloodstream but also that a physiologically appropriate amount of water will accompany that salt. ORS will therefore expand plasma volume in a highly effective way. You will remember the point above that only some of the dietary salt you eat will end up boosting blood volume: the rest is either excreted or ends up causing havoc in other parts of the body. With ORS, *this does not happen*. The salt only goes into the bloodstream, nowhere else. Therefore, ORS allows you to boost blood volume without the complicated and potentially deleterious effects of a more conventional high dietary salt intake. In this way drinking ORS is somewhat akin to having a 'Saline IV in your pocket'. The effect is, of course, not long-lasting. The kidneys will work to excrete the salty solution but the beneficial effect will last for at least a few hours and can then be repeated by the further drinking of ORS.

Indeed, ORS may be more effective than a saline IV in some ways. A most insightful recent study by Medow et al. compared the effect of ORS with saline IV for reducing orthostatic intolerance in POTS patients ('The Benefits of Oral Rehydration Solution on Children with POTS', 2019). The research team's hypothesis was that ORS, because of the salt-glucose co-transport carrier in the gut, would prove helpful for treating hypovolemia in POTS patients. The authors write:

> 'The rapid beneficial effect of ORS may be caused by increasing blood volume given its efficacy in enhancing consistent and nearly complete fluid and salt absorption through the intestinal NA+glucose co-transport (GLUT2, symporter) carrier. The effective

enteral salt and water transport system has been employed to combat the catastrophic fluid loss of infectious diarrhea. ORS in POTS may temporarily correct the central hypovolemia that has been reported in many subsets of patients with orthostatic intolerance and various types of syncope.'

Participants, who were aged between 15 and 29, drank either 1 litre of ORS (as per the WHO formula with Na+ = 90 mEq/l) or received 1 litre of saline IV. Both groups had marked improvement in blood volume and cerebral blood flow while orthostatic intolerance capacities improved significantly. Interestingly, the ORS group had greater orthostatic capacity than those who received the saline infusion (saline group orthostatic index at baseline: 100 ± 9.7 vs (post saline) 134.5 ± 17.4 / ORS group orthostatic index at baseline: 100±9.7 vs (post ORS) 155.6 ± 15.6). On the basis of their findings, Medow et al. concluded:

'Giving ORS to POTS patients produced effective, short-term mitigation of their orthostatic intolerance presumably by facilitating rapid repletion of salt and water. Within the short time course of this investigation, ORS was at least as effective in decreasing orthostatic intolerance than IV saline. This supports the use of ORS as an easy, safe practical therapy to mitigate symptoms associated with chronic orthostatic intolerance. Because ORS is inexpensive, safe and easily administered, it may be considered as an effective alternative to saline for rapid resolution of symptoms associated with orthostatic intolerance.'

Given that the improvement of orthostatic intolerance in this study is essentially due to the improvement of hypovolemia, we can justifiably conclude that ORS could also prove a safe and effective treatment for hypovolemic thirst as well. Indeed, for its convenience, safety and inexpensiveness, it should arguably be the first line of treatment.

But how much ORS should a patient drink? In my view, I think that patients suffering from hypovolemic thirst should *only* drink ORS for the most part. It should essentially replace pure water consumption. This is because any pure water that a patient drinks will, in the process of being filtered and then excreted by the kidneys, pull out some salt with it. In order to obtain the most consistent blood volume boosting effect, drinking ORS alone is likely the most effective solution. That is not to say that a cup of herbal tea or a decaf coffee here or there should pose a problem, or that there might not be times when drinking normal water might be appropriate, but I believe that the most logical method of counteracting hypovolemic thirst is to ensure that the majority of fluids consumed are also boosting plasma volume.

This suggestion also stems from my own personal experience. Indeed, in the two and a half years since my hospital stay, I have conducted various experiments to see what works best to quench my thirst. Initially, I drank around 600ml of ORS per day, raising this to 1 litre on bad days, along with increasing my dietary salt to between 8-12 grams per day. This certainly produced a better situation than my previous severe polydipsia but, over time, the effects of the increased dietary salt caused their own problems. I suffered from a certain sense of 'drying out' and I also sensed that my blood flow was worsening, including to my brain. I wondered if this was caused by the vasoconstrictive effect of the salt (as mentioned above, a meal with just four grams of salt is capable of reducing postprandial vasodilation by 50%).[106] My mood became quite low and I sometimes felt confused and disoriented. I then read up more about the research into the various effects of salt and wondered if my high intake was causing my problems. I also read the above-mentioned study into salt consumption in hunter gatherer groups, noting that this was typically less than 2.5 grams daily. Once I learnt that the salt in ORS

106. Dickinson, 'Endothelial function is impaired after a high-salt meal in healthy subjects', 2019.

is handled very differently by the body in that it purely boosts blood volume by ending up, in its entirety, in the bloodstream, I decided to try a new experiment: lower my dietary salt intake to a more moderate level while only essentially drinking ORS. This I found to work very well. Once my salt intake was down to around 4-5 grams daily, my thinking became sharper and I naturally felt calmer and happier. Meanwhile, I could feel the effect of the ORS expanding my blood volume, without any of the deleterious effects of a high dietary salt intake. It is this combination, of moderate dietary salt, along with drinking 2.5 – 3 litres of ORS every day, that has had the overall most helpful effect on my thirst. I do have the occasional decaf coffee or cup of normal water but the vast majority of my fluid intake comes from ORS. I should mention that I also tried to lower my dietary salt even further, to less than 2.5 grams daily while only drinking ORS and, while there were some benefits from this, my thirst did increase significantly and I found myself craving salt. Therefore, it seemed that the addition of some dietary salt remained an important treatment, alongside the drinking of ORS.

An Example of ORS: Normalyte

For those unfamiliar with ORS, it may be helpful to consider one such product in more detail. Normalyte was developed specifically with POTS patients in mind and in conjunction with advice from Dysautonomia International, a charity which fundraises and advocates for POTS patients (for more information, see: www.dysautonomiainternational.org). As such, the product avoids using artificial sweeteners, colours, dyes or preservatives. Interestingly, from correspondence with the company, I learnt that Normalyte was possibly the product that was used in the Medow study mentioned above.

Each pack, when dissolved in 500ml of water, contains: Sodium, 37 mEq (862mg); Potassium, 10mEq (393mg); Chloride 27 mEq; Anhydrous Dextrose, 37 mEq (6.75 grams); Citrate, 20 mEq (0.25 grams).

If a patient drinks, say, 1 litre of Normalyte, by how much will their plasma volume increase? Or, in other words, how much of the fluid they drink will be retained in the bloodstream, at least for a temporary period? Of course, initially the whole litre will be transferred into the bloodstream, but I am referring to the salty solution that may remain in the plasma, at least for a period. I believe that no clear answer to this question exists but to make my best educated guess, it would seem to me that drinking 1 litre of Normalyte will temporarily increase plasma volume by just under 500ml. This is because, at 1.724 grams of sodium, there are around 4.3 grams of salt equivalent in 1 litre of Normalyte, an amount which is essentially half the amount of salt as exists in one litre of blood. How long this effect might last for would need to be determined by future research. I imagine that the effect is rather temporary, albeit enough to provide relief, and needs to be maintained by the continuous drinking of ORS throughout the day.

While I believe, based on my own personal experience, that switching to drinking primarily ORS, along with an otherwise moderate intake of salt, may represent the best approach to dealing with hypovolemic thirst, there are a range of further options which should also be discussed. In this case, the options are medical in nature and my discussion of them comes with the caveat that my knowledge in this case is very much that of a layman. I also do not have much personal experience with these options. It could be that they represent even more effective means of counteracting the problem of hypovolemic thirst but this is not something that I am best placed to determine.

Medical Approaches to Treating Hypovolemic Dehydration

In addition to ORS, there exist various conventional medical options.

One obvious treatment could be a regular saline IV, a procedure whereby plasma volume is expanded steadily by infusion of a saline solution. Interestingly, this is a procedure which is known to benefit

POTS patients.[107] Such a procedure, on a weekly basis, would likely manage the symptoms of hypovolemic dehydration very well. However, its effects are short-lived and it is something of a hassle, for both patients and medical providers, to organise such a treatment on an ongoing basis. Furthermore, there is always the risk of infection from such IV procedures. When we consider the findings of Medow's study above, that ORS is in some ways more effective than a saline IV at improving hypovolemia, one would wonder at the wisdom of choosing an invasive procedure when such a simple, and safe, option also exists.

There are also various medications that could be useful.

The first of these is Flurinef, a synthetic form of aldosterone, the body's primary salt-retention hormone. As we saw in chapter two, aldosterone levels tend to be significantly lower in ME/CFS patients when compared to healthy controls. The use of Flurinef is a treatment with a long history in ME/CFS albeit with variable results,[108] while in POTS more obviously positive results have been reported.[109] Treatment with Flurinef needs to be done under the care of an experienced doctor and requires close monitoring of side-effects and potassium levels. I have never tried Flurinef myself although my aldosterone levels tend to be in the lower third, or once slightly below the lowest point, of the expected reference range, which is what one would expect to see in ME/CFS patients.[110] Given that increasing the body's capacity to retain salt will also thereby increase plasma volume, Flurinef could represent a highly effective means of combatting hypovolemic thirst.

107. Ruzieh et al., 'Effects of intermittent intravenous saline infusions in patients with medication-refractory postural tachycardia syndrome', 2017.

108. See a summary of relevant research here: https://sacfs.asn.au/news/2010/07/07_29_fludrocortisone_for_cfs.htm

109. Freitas et al., 'Clinical improvement in patients with orthostatic intolerance after treatment with bisoprolol and fludrocortisone', 2000.

110. Miwa, 'Down-regulation of renin-aldosterone and antidiuretic hormone systems in patients with myalgic encephalomyelitis/chronic fatigue syndrome', 2016.

The second primary medication is Desmopressin, a synthetic form of vasopressin/antidiuretic hormone. This is the mainstay of treating Diabetes Insipidus but it has also been shown to be effective in ME/CFS[111] and it is sometimes recommended as a treatment option for patients with that condition.[112] Due to RAA axis and HPA axis suppression, vasopressin also tends to be downregulated in ME/CFS and this downregulation does play a secondary role in maintaining the ongoing hypovolemic state. Desmopressin treatment could, therefore, be helpful in managing hypovolemic dehydration. However, monitoring fluid intake is critical while on Desmopressin as excessive drinking can result in hyponatraemia. As with Flurinef, this treatment requires skilful monitoring by an experienced physician. I did take Desmopressin for symptomatic relief at night, along with water restriction, in the months prior to my hospitalisation. At that time, I didn't really have any clue as to why I was suffering from such extreme thirst. The most I knew was that vasopressin output is lowered in ME/CFS and, for that reason, I had asked my doctor for a Desmopressin prescription. I came to take a third of a 120mcg sublingual pill at night. It usually had a delightful effect: I would feel my extremities become warmer as my blood volume expanded and my thirst would diminish. However, on a couple of occasions when I was more severely ill, the Desmopressin did not reduce my thirst. I'm not sure why that was the case but it created a particularly dangerous scenario and may have contributed to the very low blood sodium level that was found at the start of my hospitalisation in January 2021. In the last two and a half years, I have only taken a small amount of Desmopressin on around 15-20 occasions and hardly at all since I switched to drinking pretty much just ORS. I am naturally wary of the dangers of hyponatraemia and, while

---

111. *Ibid.*

112. See: 'ME/CFS Treatment Recommendations US ME/CFS Clinician Coalition, Version 1, February 20, 2021' (https://mecfscliniciancoalition.org/wp-content/uploads/2021/05/MECFS-Clinician-Coalition-Treatment-Recs-V1.pdf)

I did feel better on Desmopressin, I appreciate the safety of ORS which I find effective and in general well suited to my situation. Also, when one considers that the primary issue is likely that of RAA axis suppression, taking Desmopressin would seem to me to be less obviously indicated.

Finally, another possible avenue of treatment might concern efforts to increase red blood cell (RBC) volume whether in addition to, or instead of, plasma volume. This book has tended towards discussing the diminution of plasma volume. However, as noted in the previous chapter, lowered RBC volume has also been found in both ME/CFS and POTS patients. Treatment with erythropoietin, the hormone that controls red blood cell volume production might also therefore be worth considering. Indeed, a 2012 study, looking at the use of erythropoietin in POTS patients, found that 27 of 39 patients reported a sustained improvement in their orthostatic intolerance at the 6 month mark.[113] In addition, as noted in the last chapter, B12 has a role in the creation of red blood cells and could be a helpful supplement for patients with hypovolemic thirst.

Whether Flurinef, Desmopressin, Erythropoietin, or perhaps using all three simultaneously, should be the primary medical treatment for hypovolemic dehydration remains an open question. If the general thesis presented in this book is correct, the exact protocols that can best manage hypovolemic thirst remain to be determined. All medications come with side-effects, however, and those associated with Flurinef and Desmopressin in particular are not insignificant. Not only do they risk, in the one case, dangerously low potassium levels and, in the other, dangerously low sodium levels, the long-term suppression of the body's natural hormonal cycles is arguably not a good idea. In my own view, ORS represents the safest possible option but, if treatment with medication

---

113.   Kanjwal et al., 'Erythropoietin in the treatment of postural orthostatic tachy-cardia syndrome', 2012.

proved more effective and could be managed safely, then it might ultimately prove a better course of action, at least for some patients.

Concluding Thoughts on Treatment Options

All of the above suggestions obviously come with the caveat that I am not a medical professional, although I am someone who necessarily has had to spend a lot of time researching and reflecting on so-called 'Primary Polydipsia'. If hypovolemic dehydration really is a new kind of polydipsia, and one which has been psychologised erroneously, experienced medical researchers will be able to work out, much better than I can, the best course of action for treating it. However, the above suggestions seem to me to be sensible starting points and ORS in particular is likely to represent the neatest solution to daily management of the condition alongside patient education.

However, it is important for physicians to realise, if I am correct that hypovolemic dehydration exists as one part of larger more complex illnesses such as ME/CFS and POTS, that they will need to ascertain if their patients also have one of those illnesses. It seems unlikely that hypovolemic thirst exists in isolation and, as any ME/CFS patient will tell you, their thirst gets worse when they physically overextend and experience PEM (Post-Exertional Malaise). This is likely the case because, as we have explored previously, all of the central mechanisms within the illness, including RAA axis suppression, become worse during such episodes and solute loss will increase. Therefore, a crucial treatment for hypovolemic dehydration is likely to be pacing and the avoidance of Post-Exertional Malaise.

Another consideration is that physicians should review all current supplements/medications that a patient is taking in order to ensure that they are not taking anything that might worsen their hypovolemia. For example, ME/CFS patients are often recommended to take magnesium for its role in the Krebs cycle and ATP production. However, magnesium also pulls sodium out of the body and has an inhibitory effect on aldosterone, angiotensin II and renin production.[114] In my own view, it is a supplement that hypovolemic patients might be best advised to avoid. I do wonder if it contributed to my worst episodes of thirst and urination (from August 2020 – January 2021) at which point I was typically taking 500mg of magnesium daily, a supplement that I later stopped taking altogether when I learnt of its potentially negative role in the RAA axis. There can also be dietary factors, like caffeine, that increase fluid loss, as well as medications which might induce hyponatraemia: all such things should also be discussed with the patient.

It should also be mentioned that, if a patient is drinking significant amounts of ORS on a daily basis, they should probably avoid stopping their intake abruptly. This is because their body will have become accustomed to the easy supply of electrolytes and will probably struggle to adapt to a sudden shortfall. Indeed, a sudden cessation of drinking ORS could result in some kind of hypovolemic crisis. If a patient did wish to cease taking ORS, tapering off slowly would probably be the best strategy.

Is it possible to quench hypovolemic thirst completely? In my own experience, the answer is 'yes'. However, my thirst will still increase commensurately to flare-ups in my illness. At such times, I still experience excessive thirst but the intensity is typically between 10-25% of the previous nightmare that I went through and now I have the knowledge to manage the situation differently. I also think that, while hypovolemic dehydration is probably the main reason for excessive thirst in ME/CFS and related illnesses, it might not be the only reason. For example, some patients might also experience a light 'thirst sensation' in the mouth, perhaps due to less acetylcholine or some other kind of neurological dysregulation, although this will be separate from the body's actual

---

114.   Ichihara et al., 'Effects of magnesium on the renin-angiotensin-aldosterone system in human subjects', 1993.

(osmotic or volemic) hydration status.[115] In addition fluctuations in dopamine, norepinephrine, histamine, among other compounds or the excessive release of the dipsogen bradykinin (a key aspect within the hypothesis of Scheibenbogen and Wirth, as explored in chapter two) all might also contribute to increased thirst in the illness. ME/CFS patients often say that they feel very dry and there may be several reasons for that. In addition, there might also exist some kind of inflammatory processes, particularly during post-exertional malaise, that might create a temporary increase of thirst. However, ultimately, I would imagine that the most pressing reason for an *extreme* form of thirst in ME/CFS must stem from the physiological catastrophe that is hypovolemia. Despite this, however, it is feasible that even if a patient only drinks Oral Rehydration Solution, they may still struggle to quench their hypovolemic thirst fully. This is because ORS will only increase plasma volume but will have no effect on red blood cell volume which may remain low. It may be the case that the ability to tolerate a slight thirst is therefore important, at least at times. Ultimately, the full resolution of this symptom may depend upon the resolution of the underlying illness. In the main, however, it is likely that primarily drinking ORS should prove a generally effective strategy for managing hypovolemic dehydration.

---

115. For factors that might create a 'thirst sensation', see Carroll H., 'Redefining thirst: a conceptual four-compartment model characterising types of thirst, and their underlying mechanisms and interactions', 2020.

Conclusion

I have presented my case for reconsidering the symptoms of so-called Primary Polydipsia as really being driven by hypovolemic thirst. In doing so, we reviewed the early history of Primary Polydipsia, seeing that it was always subject to a strong bias towards psychologization, and that the earliest conceptions of the condition have, with some changes around the edges, remained largely ossified to this day. In line with this, we also saw how the early limits placed on understanding the condition, by considering the symptoms purely from within the lens of osmotic thirst, created a set of diagnostic procedures that were necessarily incapable of capturing the real problem. Then, we explored in detail the concept of hypovolemic thirst and how a patient with hypovolemia could easily, through mistakenly but understandably drinking pure water in response to their thirst, enter a vicious cycle and, as a result, suffer from the same clinical features that are characteristic of so-called Primary Polydipsia: very dilute urine with a tendency towards hyponatraemia. We then considered a patient population which may have always been historically misdiagnosed with Primary Polydipsia, those with ME/CFS and POTS, due to the endogenous hypovolemia that underpins their illnesses. Reasons for that hypovolemia were explored, focussing in particular on the RAA axis suppression. Previous research into Primary Polydipsia that may unwittingly support my hypothesis was also discussed and, in doing so, we found that RAA axis downregulation and resulting solute loss were elements that have likely already been identified, albeit without follow-up research to explore the implications of such findings. We considered then the considerable evidence of ME/CFS patients themselves in describing their symptoms of extreme thirst before, finally in the last chapter, suggesting possible ways of treating hypovolemic dehydration both in a hospital setting and on a day to day basis.

In the first half of this final chapter, I would like to consider possible challenges to my ideas. In particular, I will discuss whether any of the various current diagnostic procedures, namely the use copeptin, hypertonic saline infusion and the water deprivation test, could still produce results that might somehow invalidate my hypothesis. Then, I will discuss whether two prominent Primary Polydipsia subtypes, Dipsogenic Diabetes Insipidus and Primary Polydipsia as it occurs in Schizophrenia, subtypes which I have not focussed on so far in this book, could also be considered forms of hypovolemic dehydration or whether their particular characteristics deny such a possibility. With these various challenges considered, I will then, in the second half of the chapter, outline what kinds of research questions could validate my ideas before finally bringing everything together with some final, concluding remarks.

Objections

It is important to consider whether any of the current diagnostic tests used to diagnose Primary Polydipsia could also produce results that might invalidate my ideas. Might this be the case with the water deprivation test, the use of copeptin or of hypertonic saline?

To consider the first of these, if the water deprivation test demonstrates intact vasopressin function, could this be seen as having implications not just for the body's water retention capabilities but also for its blood retention capabilities? After all, the ability to retain water is one aspect of the ability to retain blood. If the body was always capable of retaining water, was it also always capable of retaining blood? But this is to forget that the primary dysfunction concerns the suppression of the RAA axis and has rather little to do with vasopressin release. Indeed, the capacity of the body to release vasopressin is largely irrelevant to my hypothesis. The sequence of events is as follows:

> RAA axis suppression >>> increased solute loss >>> lowered blood volume >>> hypovolemic thirst activated >>> mistaken drinking of high volumes of water >>> vasopressin release suppressed due to high water intake

The kicking back into action of vasopressin function due to a water deprivation test, therefore, is simply correcting the last aspect in that sequence of events. Vasopressin function was always intact (albeit likely somewhat blunted). Instead, it was majorly suppressed due to the patient's misplaced attempt to solve their legitimate problem by drinking so much water. A positive water deprivation test result, therefore, tells us nothing about the functionality of the real problem, namely the RAA axis downregulation. Similarly, the capacity of the body to self-resolve a hyponatraemic state during water deprivation will primarily stem from the steady loss of water in the urine rather than an improvement in RAA axis function.

Let us consider, secondly, the administration of hypertonic saline, a test which involves infusing a patient with a 2.5% saline solution. The rationale for doing so is to raise the internal osmotic pressure, essentially dehydrating the patient and ascertain if their body can release vasopressin in order to dilute the blood and counteract that dehydration. But even if this result is obtained, we are again told nothing about the patient's RAA axis but only about vasopressin-related functions.

Finally, in the case of copeptin testing, its supposed value relates not only to its 1:1 co-release with vasopressin but to its far more stable nature. Vasopressin is highly unstable and degrades within minutes. Copeptin, on the other hand, remains stable at room temperature for 7 days, making it a highly reliable surrogate means of testing for the quantity of vasopressin in a blood sample. Regardless of its usefulness, however, this is also purely a test of osmotic physiology and its results necessarily shed no light on RAA axis function or blood volume either.

All of these tests suffer from the original error of framing the condition purely in terms of osmotic thirst. They are akin to examining a patient's elbow bone, finding it to be intact and therefore declaring that all is well, while that patient is actually suffering from a broken leg and screaming in agony.

Having considered these diagnostic procedures, let us now turn to the two aforementioned, prominent subtypes. Can they withstand the concept of hypovolemic dehydration or might they also be, when considered in a new light, driven by that pathophysiology?

Other Primary Polydipsia Subtypes in Light of Hypovolemic Thirst: Dipsogenic Diabetes Insipidus and Primary Polydipsia in Schizophrenia

In chapter one, I reviewed various advances that have been made in the understanding of Primary Polydipsia. These included the emergence of certain subtypes, including i) a polydipsia among the 'Severe and Persistently Mentally Ill' which occurs particularly in schizophrenia and in which psychosis-driven neurological mechanisms can create hyponatraemia as well as ii) a kind of polydipsia which appears to involve solely a dysregulation in thirst mechanisms (so called 'Dipsogenic Diabetes Insipidus'). Might the idea of hypovolemic thirst shed any light on either of these problems?

Let us consider first 'Dipsogenic Diabetes Insipidus', sometimes also referred to as 'Dipsogenic Polydipsia', a condition in which the patient's thirst mechanisms have gone supposedly awry. In Goldman and Ahmadi's 2020 overview of Primary Polydipsia,[116] they suggest that this condition is 'thirst-driven with no apparent psychological factors' and entails a 'disruption of homeostatic influences on thirst'. In particular, some kind of thirst 'reset osmostat' seems to be at play such that patients exhibit a 'low osmotic threshold for thirst'. In addition to this, the other defining feature is a 'relative increased threshold' for vasopressin release or, in other words, as the blood stream becomes more concentrated, triggering dehydration, vasopressin is not released as soon as one would expect in order to conserve water. As a result of these two factors, patients with 'Dipsogenic Diabetes Insipidus' are not viewed as drinking large amounts of fluid as a result of mental ill-health. One of the first more developed descriptions of the condition was by Robertson in 1987 in an article entitled 'Dipsogenic diabetes insipidus: a newly recognized syndrome caused by a selective defect in the osmoregulation of thirst'. In that article, which was based on his observations of just three patients, Robertson admitted that the 'pathogenesis of the osmoregulatory abnormality is unknown but may be due to disruption of one or more of the afferent pathways that regulate the "set" of the thirst and vasopressin osmostats'.

While it is feasible that 'dipsogenic diabetes insipidus' stems from some kind of thirst dysregulation of as yet unknown origin, its two central characteristics, namely of a low osmotic thirst threshold and of a high release point for vasopressin, could also accord entirely with the idea of hypovolemic dehydration. In the case of the low osmotic thirst threshold, this could simply be a misreading of the situation. For, if you were unaware that the real reason for a patient's constant thirst was their hypovolemia, and if you therefore remained purely tied to considering thirst from an osmotic perspective, then you could naturally conclude that the thirst threshold of a patient who is seemingly 'drinking

---

116. Goldman and Ahmadi, 'Primary polydipsia: update', 2020.

too much, too soon' must have been reset downwards. In truth, the osmotic set point for thirst is utterly irrelevant to this patient's problem. Their thirst centre hasn't been 'reset downwards' at all. Rather, it is a completely different thirst centre that is driving the drinking. In such a scenario in which the hypovolemia remains constant, the drinking will always occur well before the body's true needs from an osmotic thirst perspective, thus deceiving the observer into concluding that a lowered osmotic thirst threshold has been created. The idea of a 'low osmotic thirst threshold', therefore, could be nothing other than the product of looking at the problem from the wrong angle.

The second key characteristic of 'Dipsogenic Diabetes Insipidus', namely the higher threshold for vasopressin release, can also be explained in light of this book's hypothesis. Indeed, the general downregulation of the RAA and HPA axes will usually also blunt the release of vasopressin. As Miwa showed in his 2016 paper, vasopressin levels in ME/CFS patients are significantly lower than in controls.[117] Therefore, the observation that vasopressin has a 'higher release threshold' could simply result from looking at a blunted-vasopressin response also from the wrong perspective.

A final consideration is that the use of Desmopressin is often recommended in cases of 'Dipsogenic Diabetes Insipidus' and usually leads to symptomatic improvement. But could this improvement primarily stem from the drug's role as a volume expander? Towards the end of chapter two, we considered a 1983 case study by Mellinger in which a patient with a supposed thirst-dysregulation responded very well to Desmopressin. In the case of that patient, her intake, while on Desmopressin, was 2.5 litres while her output was just 875 ml, indicating a significant internal volume increase. Was this the real reason for her clinical improvement?

---

117. Miwa, 'Down-regulation of renin-aldosterone and antidiuretic hormone systems in patients with myalgic encephalomyelitis/chronic fatigue syndrome', 2016.

I am not best placed to know whether the condition that is currently termed 'Dipsogenic Diabetes Insipidus' is simply a mistaken snapshot of various aspects of hypovolemic dehydration but it seems to me that its central features can be explained by reference to a hypovolemia-driven thirst. A future research study that examined the blood volume status of patients diagnosed specifically with 'Dipsogenic Diabetes Insipidus' would certainly be well placed to find out one way or the other.

Let us now turn to the other major subtype within Primary Polydipsia, namely Primary Polydipsia as it occurs in patients with severe mental ill-health and with schizophrenia in particular. Indeed, I will limit my discussion to Primary Polydipsia as it occurs in schizophrenia because it seems, from reading the medical literature, that it is schizophrenia in which, of all psychiatric conditions, so-called Primary Polydipsia seems to co-exist by far the most. Whether the ideas presented here have any relevance for excessive thirst in other serious mental health conditions, I will leave it to more expert minds than my own to decide. In any event, can hypovolemic dehydration also shed light on so-called Primary Polydipsia in schizophrenic patients?

The short answer is that, while I am not well placed to make any strong suggestions one way or another, I do think that there might be some surprising reasons to regard the concept of hypovolemic dehydration as offering an explanation for excessive thirst and fluid consumption, at least among some schizophrenic patients.

I would never even have thought to consider such a possibility until I came across research that posits a strong possible link between ME/CFS and schizophrenia. Indeed, similarities between the two conditions are presented in a series of recent papers by Kanchanatawan et al. and it is worth mentioning their titles for greater context. They are: i) 'In schizophrenia, chronic fatigue syndrome- and fibromyalgia-like symptoms are driven by breakdown of the paracellular pathway with increased zonulin and immune activation-associated neurotoxicity' (2023), ii) 'Chronic fatigue syndrome and fibromyalgia-like symptoms are an integral component of the phenome of schizophrenia: neuro-immune and opioid system correlates' (2020) and iii) 'Chronic fatigue and fibromyalgia symptoms are key components of deficit schizophrenia and are strongly associated with activated immune-inflammatory pathways' (2020).

In reaching their conclusions, Kanchanatawan at al. measured, in the second study just mentioned, various markers associated with neurotoxic immune pathways and lowered immune regulation in schizophrenic patients (these pathophysiological mechanisms are typical of ME/CFS as well). The authors also asked these patients to complete a 'fibro-fatigue' scale in which ME- and Fibromyalgia-related symptoms are measured. The results showed that the higher the fibro-fatigue (FF) scores, the more pronounced were various schizophrenic symptoms. The authors write: 'Patients with an increased FF score display increased ratings of psychosis, hostility, excitement, formal thought disorders, psycho-motor retardation and negative symptoms as compared with patients with lower FF scores.' It was also found that the various blood markers for neurotoxicity and lowered immune regulation correlated with the fibro-fatigue scores. In the third study mentioned above, Kanchanatawan et al. further found that patients with 'deficit schizophrenia', namely a kind of schizophrenia that is characterised by more 'negative' symptoms, have a particularly strong correlation with ME- and Fibromyalgia-like symptoms. In that study, it was found that in patients with deficit schizophrenia, 'there were robust associations between FF and negative symptoms, psychosis, hostility, excitation, mannerism, psychomotor retardation and formal thought disorders', and that these symptoms were strongly correlated with immune system dysregulation and increased cytokine production. Finally, the first-mentioned study above conducted by Kanchanatawan et al. examined other ME-related pathophysiological mechanisms within schizophrenia patients, including zonulin levels (a marker for 'leaky gut'), immune IgM related dysregulation and increased levels of tryptophan catabolites. That study reached similar conclusions, stating: 'It is concluded that FF symptoms are part of the phenome schizophrenia and BCPS [behavioural-cognitive-physical-psychosocial]-worsening as well.'

These studies left me very curious to know more. If schizophrenia and ME/CFS share certain similarities in terms of neurotoxicity and immune dysregulation, could they also share other pathophysiological dysfunctions? And, most relevant of all to this book's hypothesis, might some schizophrenics also suffer from low blood volume and could, therefore, their thirst be explained on that account? And what about vasopressin and the RAA axis in schizophrenia?

While there is very little research that has considered these kinds of questions, there is one paper, published all the way back in 1938 by Finkelman and Haffron, that brought me up short. Titled 'Observations on the Circulating Blood Volume in Schizophrenia, Manic-Depressive Psychosis, Epilepsy, Involutional Psychosis and Mental Deficiency', the results of its research, despite being conducted over 80 years ago, have potentially very significant implications for this book's hypothesis. Due to a technical error, I was unfortunately unable to purchase the original article, but its most pertinent findings were summarised in the year after its publication by G.W.T.H. Fleming as follows:

'The writers found a low circulating blood volume in patients with schizophrenia, as compared with manic-depressive patients, whose circulating blood volume approaches normal. The schizophrenics had a blood volume per square metre of body surface of 2,609 c.c., as compared with 2,973 c.c. in manic-depressive patients. The plasma volume in schizophrenia per square metre of body surface was 1,433 c.c., as compared with 1,727 c.c. in the manic-depressive patients. The diminution in the circulating blood volume in schizophrenia appears to be related to disturbances in water metabolism, capillary permeability and vasomotor tonus, secretion of the antidiuretic and vasopressor hormone of the posterior pituitary gland, basal oxygen consumption rate and indirectly heat regulation. These failings may be due to dysfunction of the hypothalamus. The circulating blood volume in involutional psychoses was lower than in schizophrenia.'[118]

At 2,609 c.c. per square metre, these schizophrenics had a total blood volume reduction of around 12.5% in comparison to the more normal amount that was found in the manic-depressives while, in terms of plasma volume, the reduction was even more profound at around 20%. On such a basis, these schizophrenics had, like many ME/CFS patients, experienced a plasma blood volume drop well past the 10% that is required to trigger the hypovolemic thirst centre. Was this blood volume drop because of something specific to schizophrenia? Or did these patients also have ME/CFS and therefore experience hypovolemia only as part of having that illness as a comorbidity? Or is it because schizophrenia and ME/CFS may, at least in some cases, manifest very similarly? In addition, albeit from a position of medical science in 1938, one cannot help but note that the reasons given for the blood volume drop, as described by Fleming, are rather similar to some of the general dysfunctions seen within ME/CFS.

Having read about this extraordinary study, I searched, almost entirely in vain, to find any similar and more recent studies into blood volume among schizophrenics: perhaps its supposedly psychiatric basis has resulted in a general lack of interest in endocrine abnormalities in the condition. I did, however, come across a study looking at blood volume specifically within the brain of schizophrenic patients. Written by Brambilla et al. in 2007 and with the title 'Assessment of cerebral blood volume in schizophrenia: A magnetic resonance imaging study', the paper found that schizophrenics do indeed have lower blood volume in the

---

118. G.W.T.H. Fleming, *Journal of Mental Science*, 1938.

brain. The authors concluded: 'Hypothetically, chronic low CBV [cerebral blood volume] may sustain neural hypoactivation and concomitant increase of free radicals, ultimately resulting in neuronal loss and cognitive impairments. Thus, altered intracranial hemodynamics may accompany brain atrophy and cognitive deficits, being a crucial factor in the pathophysiology of schizophrenia.' But if there is less blood in the brain, it is surely not too much of a leap to conclude that there will be less blood everywhere else in the body also and, in this way, this far more recent study adds further evidence to the possibility of a hypovolemic thirst also existing in schizophrenia.

From here, I tried to find research into RAA axis function in schizophrenia as well as possible diminutions in antidiuretic hormone. Regarding the latter, I came across three studies that showed vasopressin is lower in schizophrenic patients in comparison with healthy controls[119] while regarding the former, I found one particularly relevant study (Mohite et al., 'Lower circulating levels of angiotensin-converting enzyme (ACE) in patients with schizophrenia', 2018). This paper looked closely at RAA axis function within 25 patients with schizophrenia and 20 controls. The results showed a clear trend towards lower angiotensin-converting enzyme but no real difference in plasma levels of ACE2, angiotensin (Ang)-(1-7) and, crucially, angiotensin II (missing, also, were measurements of renin and of aldosterone). I do not know exactly how these results might correlate with the expected pattern in ME/CFS or POTS but I would imagine that the latter conditions should also involve an obviously lowered production of angiotensin II, given its more critical role in maintaining salt and water balance. Nevertheless, this paper does clearly further support the idea that there could be some sort of

119. Sarai and Matsunaga, 'ADH secretion in schizophrenic patients on antipsychotic drugs', 1989; 'Rubin et al., 'Reduced Levels of Vasopressin and Reduced Behavioural Modulation of Oxytocin in Psychotic Disorders', 2014; Jobst et al., 'Oxytocin and vasopressin levels are decreased in the plasma of male schizophrenia patients', 2013.

RAA axis suppression in schizophrenia as well. At the very least, as its authors conclude: 'Our results corroborate the hypothesis that the RAS is involved in the pathophysiology of schizophrenia'.

When I started out writing this book, I did not imagine that my ideas would pose any real challenge to the kind of Primary Polydipsia that has been considered a subtype within schizophrenia but all of the aforementioned research has forced me to think that there is perhaps a possibility that at least some schizophrenics suffer from extreme thirst primarily due to low blood volume, just as I believe occurs in ME/CFS and related illnesses. But this possibility raises many, much larger questions: What exactly is the relationship between ME/CFS and schizophrenia? Are they the same illness, an idea that seems unlikely on the face of it, or do they rather just share certain pathophysiological mechanisms (but not most)? Or is there more overlap than one might imagine? For example, do some schizophrenic patients suffer from post-exertional malaise? If they do suffer from key ME/CFS mechanisms, then can we say that they have schizophrenia at all? Or are they rather suffering from personality and other psychological changes driven by the reduced cerebral perfusion that is so characteristic of ME/CFS? And, if that is the case, has such an illness presentation always been mislabelled as schizophrenia out of ignorance for what is really going on?

I'll leave these questions dangling in the air: I cannot possibly answer them. All I can say is that, if my ideas about hypovolemia-induced thirst in ME/CFS are correct, then blood volume status in schizophrenics with polydipsia, on the basis of the aforementioned research, clearly needs to be clarified as well. On a more anecdotal front, I will also mention that I came across a podcast by a schizophrenic patient discussing her mental health journey. In her podcast, 'Living with psychogenic polydipsia', she described her issues with extreme thirst, a symptom from which she had suffered over a long period of time. However, near the beginning of that episode, she also mentioned that she has POTS and dysautonomia as comorbidities. So why did she really have her polydipsia?[120]

On the flip side, there does seem to exist mechanisms particular to schizophrenia through which patients can develop hyponatraemia specifically during episodes of psychosis. These were described in chapter one and tend to involve, through neurological stress-related dysregulation, an inappropriately high release of vasopressin during psychosis and resultant low blood sodium. Such a mechanism does not appear to occur in ME/CFS in which vasopressin tends to be low regardless. Furthermore, ME/CFS patients in general do not have the hallmark symptoms of schizophrenia such as hallucinations, delusions, paranoia or hearing voices (although they can suffer from emotional lability, social withdrawal, a flat emotional affect and various other negative personality changes, all as a result of the effect of their biomedical illness on their neurological function). Also, some of the self-reported reasons, in May's 1995 research survey, among psychiatric inpatients regarding their high fluid consumption, such as 'the voices tell me to drink' and 'to get a high by drinking', are entirely unrelated to the typical experience of the ME/CFS patient who drinks a lot of fluid simply because of a raging thirst. In addition, 14 of the 45 patients in that study also admitted to having drunk their own urine, something that suggests strongly mental ill-health. It is quite possible therefore that schizophrenia has a kind of polydipsia that is particular to it. However this does not rule out the possibility of a second kind of polydipsia within schizophrenia that might stem from an RAA axis dysfunction that is similar to that which is observed in ME/CFS nor the possibility that some schizophrenic patients might also have ME/CFS as a comorbidity and suffer from excessive thirst purely on that account. It is relevant to remember at this point that only a minority of schizophrenics (albeit a significant

---

120. Parker R., 'Living with psychogenic polydipsia', from the podcast Psychosis Psositivity (episode released: March 28th, 2022).

one) suffer from polydipsia.[121] The fact that this is not a phenomenon witnessed among all schizophrenics implies that it is not necessarily a defining characteristic of schizophrenia *per se*. It may exist because of a dysregulation within a specific schizophrenia subset or it could occur in a schizophrenic patient because of a comorbidity, such as ME/CFS. Only further research can answer such questions. [122]

So far in this final chapter, we have looked at a range of possible objections to my hypothesis and also considered the implications of the concept of hypovolemic dehydration on two prominent subtypes of so-called Primary Polydipsia. Next, we should consider what kind of research might need to be done in order to validate the main ideas within this book.

Questions for Future Research

How can the idea of hypovolemic dehydration be confirmed?

What would be most insightful would be to take a group of symptomatic so-called Primary Polydipsia patients. Ideally, such patients would be drinking significant amounts of fluid, e.g. over 6 litres per day, indicating that their bodies really are suffering, in a more profound way, from whatever dysfunction is going on. One aim of such a study could be to measure the plasma and red blood cell volumes of the patients: do these patients have a physiologically normal amount of blood or are they deficient and, if so, by how much? Do they have at least 10%

---

121. A 2013 study by Iftene et al. ('Identification of primary polydipsia in a severe and persistent mental illness outpatient population: a prospective observational study') of 89 psychiatric outpatients found that 15.7% had Primary Polydipsia (and, of these, 90.4% has schizophrenia).

122. I have wondered whether the conclusion that increased vasopressin is released in psychotic episodes might be a misreading of suppressed RAA-axis induced solute loss. Both scenarios would result in hyponatraemia: in the first case, a more dilutional form while, in the latter, one driven significantly by solute loss. However, I have not studied the relevant papers enough to be sure of this suggestion.

less plasma volume than the physiological norm, thereby triggering the hypovolemic thirst centre? As part of such measurements, the same patients could also be tested for their RAA axis hormones (in particular: renin, angiotensin II, aldosterone). Are these hormones notably lower when compared to healthy controls? What happens to RAA axis function when these patients go on a low salt diet: does it increase appropriately or does it remain blunted? How does the RAA axis in this patient group respond to the administration of angiotensin II? Does it upregulate, as per the physiological norm, or conversely still show evidence of suppression? Erythropoietin and haematocrit could also be measured and compared to healthy controls to understand better the red blood cell volume side of the equation.

Then, the same patients could be monitored for their response to measures to boost blood volume. If all patients adopt a moderate salt intake and swap all pure water with oral rehydration solution, does their subjectively-reported thirst diminish? What is their input and output on such a regimen, in comparison to previously? If such patients are administered a saline IV, does their sensation of thirst reduce and do they report general improvement?

Finally, the larger health context of such patients should be ascertained in order to see whether they have a hypovolemic-illness. Do they experience post-exertional malaise, suggesting ME/CFS? Or do they experience tachycardia while standing, suggesting POTS? Was their ill-health triggered by a viral illness or another significant stressor?

A study with such research questions would, I believe, be more than well-placed to validate the concept of hypovolemic dehydration.

Conclusion

In 1988, Ean Proctor, a 12-year-old boy in the Isle of Man, was removed from his parents' care and moved to a psychiatric unit. He, and his parents, claimed that he had ME/CFS along with the usual devastating reactions to exercise. Ean's case was particularly severe: he was bedridden and even suffered from episodic paralysis. The relevant healthcare authorities saw his case differently, however. The boy was merely suffering from 'school phobia' and his parents were reinforcing their child's erroneous beliefs. The boy's 'treatment' included being put unsupported into a hydrotherapy pool so as to force him to exercise. Ean had such little strength that he nearly drowned and had to be saved. He was also not supported in trips to the bathroom, perhaps also to 'encourage' him to make the trip himself, with the result that he lay in his own urine-soaked clothes.[123]

What is it that makes a doctor look at patients and blame them for their suffering? And how is it that the medical profession, governments and society at large can turn a blind eye to such incidents which, if they involved patients with other illnesses, would result in widespread condemnation?

This sort of approach has its roots in Freud and related thinkers who promulgated the idea that dark subconscious forces could somehow manifest in physical symptoms. While there is of course a link between mind and body, the nature of Freudian claims belongs more to quasi-religious belief than the scientific method. Freudian ideas fall into the category of assumptions, general theories, and a kind of worldview with its own mythologies and creeds. Whatever its merits (and there are some), it should be obvious to anyone that ideas of a Freudian nature, if utilised in medical research, should also be subjected to rigorous evaluation in accordance with the scientific method, rather than accepted as fact. Even today, when Freud's legacy has dwindled somewhat, the idea that some patients may be suffering from something 'all in the mind' is still

---

123. Ean's story is summarised here: https://me-pedia.org/wiki/Ean_Proctor and is also featured in Martin Walker's 2003 book, *Skewed*: *Psychiatric Hegemony and the Manufacture of Mental Illness in Multiple Chemical Sensitivity, Gulf War Syndrome, Myalgic Encephalomyelitis and Chronic Fatigue Syndrome*.

often considered an acceptable diagnosis. It is bizarre that otherwise smart doctors trained in the importance of the scientific method should be happy to consider an evidently suffering patient in such a way rather than roll up their sleeves and try to find out what might really be going on. The result is a 'blame the victim' approach to medicine in which the ill patient is left feeling unheard, isolated and, crucially, untreated. Worse for the patient, sometimes, than the lack of medical help is that she might also become ostracized by family members who may prefer to believe the doctor's word over her own. After all, the 'experts' can't be wrong: if the doctor says that our family member, who is bedridden and fed through a gastric tube, is just suffering from hypochondria, then who are we to say otherwise?

As the now retired Dr. William Weir, formerly of the Royal Free Hospital in London, suggests, this kind of approach is rooted not in science but in dogma. In an incisive recent article, co-written with Dr. Nigel Speight and titled 'ME/CFS: Past, Present and Future', Weir discussed the historical tendency within medicine to view poorly understood symptoms in psychological terms. These included Multiple Sclerosis, complications from tertiary syphilis, Parkinson's disease and peptic ulcers, all now illnesses that are understood to have serious organic causes. For Weir, ME/CFS has suffered from the same dynamic:

> 'The story of ME/CFS is a prime example of such dogma. Due to the fact that routine laboratory tests for the diagnosis of this condition usually produce "normal" results, the problem must be with the psyche. One of the foundation stones of this dogma was a paper published in the BMJ in 1970 in which the cause of the famous Royal Free outbreak of ME/CFS in 1955 was attributed to "mass hysteria". The authors did not interview any of the patients, nor any of the doctors involved; nonetheless, it seemed clear to them that the outbreak was due to mass hysteria because the majority of victims were women. The background to this piece of sophistry

was, and remains, the fashionable medical culture of linking physical symptoms to a psychological disorder.'

It is my contention that so-called 'Primary Polydipsia' is merely yet another example of this 'fashionable medical culture of linking physical symptoms to a psychological disorder'. Indeed, it was entirely the product of an era in which such linking was common. Not only that, it was also the product of medical thinking prior to the discovery of the hypovolemic thirst centre, something that can render explicable all of its symptoms and clinical features.

So-called Primary Polydipsia urgently needs to be reconsidered, therefore, with fresh eyes: why are these patients *really* complaining of such extreme thirst? Once this re-evaluation happens then I believe that it will only be a matter of time before Primary Polydipsia, as it is currently understood, will be consigned to the medical wastebin and the concept of hypovolemic dehydration will take its place. At that point, I believe it will become clear that the only real 'craziness' in the whole debacle of so-called Primary Polydipsia was the idea that patients drinking such enormous quantities of water must have been doing so because of mental illness rather than because of an organic pathology. You really do have to let go of normal rational thought to be content with the idea that mental ill-health can explain such a phenomenon, particularly when so-called Primary Polydiptics have always said that extreme thirst is their number one reason for drinking. And when the idea of hypovolemic thirst is validated, then those who suffer from it can, at last, receive proper medical attention rather than a 'care' which, at the moment, amounts to a continuous, if unintentional, medical negligence. And, as for those few patients who do, as I mentioned in the Introduction, drink excessive water purely for psychological reasons, they should probably also be categorised differently: they do not suffer from thirst and therefore do not technically have a 'polydipsia'. They merely have a mistaken habit, for whatever reason.

Regardless of the impact of this book on Primary Polydipsia, I hope that it might also lead to research within ME/CFS and POTS into the kind of thirst that appears to occur in those affected with such illnesses along with treatment guidelines for it. Hypovolemic dehydration carries a strong risk of hyponatraemia and, therefore, cerebral oedema and death. Physicians treating ME/CFS and POTS patients need to understand the nature of this problem quickly: for some patients the excessive thirst might just be a daily nuisance but for a minority of others it might spell death. And, with the advent of Long Covid, the prevalence of this symptom is increasing exponentially, as we saw in chapter two. With around a third of Long Covid patients citing extreme thirst as one of their main symptoms, unravelling the exact mechanisms for thirst within these kinds of illnesses takes on an additional urgency. In my view, hypovolemia is likely to be the most significant reason for this excessive thirst but, as noted at the end of chapter four, it is also highly feasible that additional mechanisms contribute to the polydipsia within these illnesses. Research on thirst in these conditions would likely result in a picture that expands, most significantly, our current knowledge of thirst.

I also hope that the book will ultimately result in more awareness about ME/CFS among medical specialists from other fields. Indeed, it is the lack of general knowledge about ME/CFS that has probably resulted in the absence of any real challenging of Primary Polydipsia until now. Had it been otherwise, I imagine that the idea of hypovolemic dehydration would have been conceptualised long ago. The continued suffering of patients with so-called Primary Polydipsia therefore is almost certainly the result of the lack of interest shown by the general medical profession towards ME/CFS over decades. Primary Polydipsia was always likely to be explained by a blind spot in mainstream medical thinking and that blind spot was ME/CFS. Conversely, if the concept of hypovolemic dehydration is validated, then it could become a way in which knowledge about ME/CFS becomes widespread in the medical profession. Indeed, it would be impossible to teach medical students about hypovolemic dehydration without also teaching them about the relevant pathophysiological mechanisms within ME/CFS and POTS as well as other key findings in those illnesses thereby, in turn, ultimately leading to more interest and research. Those future medical students might well ask: why was it that we were never taught before about illnesses with such devastating pathophysiologies? They would be right to wonder.

The thirst that I experienced while suffering from my worst episodes of hypovolemic dehydration was more terrifying than I could ever convey in words. My body screamed with thirst. I was fading away, dying. I was determined that, if those were to be my last moments, I would at least die with the image of my late mother's smile in my mind. But that image also was faint and fading away.

At this very moment, there are many people who feel they are fading away from these symptoms. They need help but they receive none. They need compassion but instead the current approach implicitly mocks their suffering. Who will take it upon themselves to care for these patients at last? Who will take it upon themselves to listen to what these patients have to say? Who will take it upon themselves to banish Freud's long and cruel shadow, a shadow that has mischaracterised a real, severe and potentially fatal biomedical pathology as mental illness?

In the Introduction, I noted Prof. Daniel Bichet's words of caution about Primary Polydipsia, namely that: 'The diagnosis of compulsive water drinking must be made with care and may represent our ignorance of yet undescribed pathophysiological mechanisms.' Perhaps hypovolemic dehydration does not represent the whole story: perhaps there are other parts of the puzzle that will still remain to be unravelled. But, from everything that I have read in the medical literature and from reflecting on this question over a long time, I do believe strongly that those 'yet undescribed pathophysiological mechanisms' are driven by hypovolemic dehydration.

List of Abbreviations Used

ACE – Angiotensin Converting Enzyme

ADH – Anti-Diuretic Hormone (aka: Vasopressin & AVP – Arginine Vasopressin)

ANF – Atrial Natriuretic Factor

ATP – Adenosine Triphosphate

DI – Diabetes Insipidus

EPO – Erythropoietin

FF – Fibro-Fatigue (Scale)

FM – Fibromyalgia

hEDS – Hypermobile Ehlers Danlos Syndrome

HPA axis – Hypothalamus-Pituitary-Adrenal Axis

KKS – Kallikrein-Kinin System

MCAS – Mast Cell Activation Syndrome

ME/CFS – Myalgic Encephalomyelitis / Chronic Fatigue Syndrome

OCD – Obsessive Compulsive Disorder

OI – Orthostatic Intolerance

ORS – Oral Rehydration Solution

PEM – Post-Exertional Malaise

POTS – Postural Orthostatic Tachycardia Syndrome

RAA Axis – Renin-Angiotensin-Aldosterone Axis

RBC volume – Red Blood Cell volume

SPMI – Severely & Persistently Mentally Ill

Acknowledgements

I wish to thank my dear friend, mentor and former Irish teacher, Garry Bannister, for his thoughtful comments on an earlier draft of this book.

I also wish to thank other dear friends for their support, advice and for regularly making my day with our correspondences and conversations: Catriona, Karen, Jenny, Lauren, Fiona, Richard & Char.

I thank my Dad for his regularly stimulating conversations and for providing a refuge in these last few, rather unusual years.

Finally, I wish to thank Dr. Robin Satanovskij and Nurse Lisa from Bayreuth Dialyse Centrum, Germany, for their HELP apheresis treatments that improved my health earlier this year.

Bibliography

Aguree and Gernand, 'Plasma volume expansion across healthy pregnancy: a systematic review and meta-analysis of longitudinal studies', *BMC Pregnancy Childbirth*, 2019.

Arai et al., 'Thirst in critically ill patients: from physiology to sensation', *The American Journal of Critical Care*, 2013.

Barlow and De Wardener., 'Compulsive water drinking', *Quarterly Journal of Medicine*, 1959.

Baudrand et al., 'High sodium intake is associated with increased gluco-corticoid production, insulin resistance and metabolic syndrome', *Clinical Endocrinology*, 2014.

Bhatia et al., 'Psychogenic Polydipsia – Management Challenges', *Shanghai Archives of Psychiatry*, 2017.

Bichet DG, 'Chapter 8 - The Posterior Pituitary' in Melmed S, Ed. *The Pituitary (4th Edition)*, 2017.

Bramante et al., 'Outpatient treatment of Covid-19 with metformin, ivermectin, and fluvoxamine and the development of Long Covid over 10-month follow up', *The Lancet*, 2022.

Brambilla et al., 'Assessment of cerebral blood volume in schizophrenia: A magnetic resonance imaging study', *Journal of Psychiatric Research*, 2007.

Campbell et al., 'Proposed Nomenclature for Salt Intake and for Reductions in Dietary Salt', *The Journal of Clinical Hypertension*, 2015.

Chadda et al., 'Long COVID-19 and Postural Orthostatic Tachycardia Syndrome- Is Dysautonomia to Be Blamed?', *Frontiers in Cardiovascular Medicine*, 2022.

Carroll H., 'Redefining thirst: a conceptual four-compartment model characterising types of thirst, and their underlying mechanisms and interactions', *NutriXiv Preprints*, 2020.

Dani et al., 'Autonomic dysfunction in "long COVID": rationale, physiology and management strategies', *Clinical Medicine Journal (Royal College of Physicians, London)*, 2021.

H.E. Davis et al., 'Characterizing long Covid in an international cohort: 7 months of symptoms and their impact', *EClinicalMedicine*, 2021.

R. Davis et al., 'A Comprehensive Examination of Severely Ill ME/CFS Patients', *Healthcare (Basel)*, 2021.

R. Davis et al., 'A nanoelectronics-blood-based diagnostic biomarker for myalgic encephalomyelitis/chronic fatigue syndrome (ME/CFS)', *Proceedings of the National Academy of Sciences of the United States of America*, 2019.

Dickinson, 'Endothelial function is impaired after a high-salt meal in healthy subjects', *The American Journal of Clinical Nutrition*, 2019.

DiNicolantonio & O'Keefe, 'Low-grade metabolic acidosis as a driver of chronic disease: a 21st century public health crisis', *Open Heart*, 2021.

Edwards and Farquhar, 'Vascular Effects of Dietary Salt', *Current Opinion in Nephrology and Hypertension*, 2015.

Faraco et al., 'Dietary salt promotes neurovascular and cognitive dysfunction through a gut-initiated TH17 response', *Nature Neuroscience*, 2018.

Farquhar et al., 'Blood volume and its relation to peak O(2) consumption and physical activity in patients with chronic fatigue', *American Journal of Physiology-Heart and Circulatory Physiology*, 2002.

Ferguson et al., 'High dietary salt-induced DC activation underlies microbial dysbiosis-associated hypertension', *Journal of Clinical Investigation*, 2019.

Fleming GWTH, 'A Note On: Observations on The Circulating Blood Volume in Schizophrenia, Manic-Depressive Psychosis, Epilepsy, Involutional Psychosis and Mental Deficiency', *Journal of Mental Science*, March 1938, p. 433.

Freitas et al., 'Clinical improvement in patients with orthostatic intolerance after treatment with bisoprolol and fludrocortisone', *Clinical Autonomic Research*, 2000.

Geisberger et al., 'Salt Transiently Inhibits Mitochondrial Energetics in Mononuclear Phagocytes', *Circulation*, 2021.

Goldman and Ahmadi, 'Primary Polydipsia: update', *Best Practice & Research Clinical Endocrinology & Metabolism*, 2020.

Goldman, 'Brain circuit dysfunction in a distinct subset of chronic psychotic patients', *Schizophrenia Research*, 2018.

Goldman et al., 'Psychotic exacerbations and enhanced vasopressin secretion in schizophrenic patients with hyponatraemia and polydipsia', *Archives of General Psychiatry*, 1997.

Han et al., 'Hyponatraemic seizure secondary to primary polydipsia following urological surgery', *BMJ Case Report*, 2022.

Hurwitz et al., 'Chronic fatigue syndrome: illness severity, sedentary lifestyle, blood volume and evidence of diminished cardiac function', *Clinical Science (London)*, 2010.

Ichihara et al., 'Effects of magnesium on the renin-angiotensin-aldosterone system in human subjects', *Journal of Laboratory and Clinical Medicine*, 1993.

Iftene et al., 'Identification of primary polydipsia in a severe and persistent mental illness outpatient population: a prospective observational study', *Psychiatry Research*, 2013.

Jobst et al., 'Oxytocin and vasopressin levels are decreased in the plasma of male schizophrenia patients', *Acta Neuropsychiatrica*, 2013.

Johnson A., 'The Sensory Psychobiology of Thirst and Salt Appetite', *Medicine & Science in Sports & Exercise (MSSE)*, 2007.

Johnson C., 'Dr. David Bell on Low Blood Volume in Chronic Fatigue Syndrome' (website: https://www.healthrising.org/forums/resources/dr-david-bell-on-low-blood-volume-in-chronic-fatigue-syndrome.234/)

Johnson C., 'Enhancing Blood Volume in Chronic Fatigue Syndrome (ME/CFS) and Fibromyalgia' (website: www.healthrising.org/treating-chronic-fatigue-syndrome/enhancing-blood-volume-in-chronic-fatigue-syndrome-mecfs-and-fibromyalgia/)

Jin-lim et al., 'Prospects of the Two-Day Cardiopulmonary Exercise Test (CPET) in ME/CFS patients: A Meta-Analysis', *Journal of Clinical Medicine*, 2020.

Kanchanatawan et al., 'In schizophrenia, chronic fatigue syndrome- and fibromyalgia-like symptoms are driven by breakdown of the paracellular pathway with increased zonulin and immune activation-associated neurotoxicity', *CNS & Neurological Disorders - Drug Targets*, 2023.

Kanchanatawan et al., 'Chronic fatigue syndrome and fibromyalgia-like symptoms are an integral component of the phenome of schizophrenia: neuro-immune and opioid system correlates', *Metabolic Brain Disease*, 2020.

Kanchanatawan et al., 'Chronic fatigue and fibromyalgia symptoms are key components of deficit schizophrenia and are strongly associated with activated immune-inflammatory pathways', *Schizophrenia Research*, 2020.

Kanjwal et al., 'Erythropoietin in the treatment of postural orthostatic tachycardia syndrome', *American Journal of Therapeutics*, 2012.

König et al., 'The Gut Microbiome in Myalgic Encephalomyelitis (ME)/ Chronic Fatigue Syndrome (CFS)', *Frontiers in Immunology*, 2021.

May DL., 'Patient perceptions of self-induced water intoxication', *Archives of Psychiatric Nursing*, 1995.

Medow et al., 'The Benefits of Oral Rehydration Solution on Children with POTS', *The Journal of Pediatrics*, 2019.

Mellinger, 'Primary polydipsia. Syndrome of inappropriate thirst', *Archives of Internal Medicine*, 1983.

Miller A.H., 'Decreased Basal Ganglia Activation in Subjects with Chronic Fatigue Syndrome: Association with Symptoms of Fatigue', *PLOS ONE*, 2014.

Miller W., 'Psychogenic Factors in the Polyuria of Schizophrenia', *Journal of Nervous and Mental Disease*, 1936.

Millson et al., 'A survey of patient attitudes toward self-induced water intoxication', *Canadian Journal of Psychiatry*, 1992.

Miwa, 'Down-regulation of renin-aldosterone and antidiuretic hormone systems in patients with myalgic encephalomyelitis/chronic fatigue syndrome', *Journal of Cardiology*, 2016.

Mohite et al., 'Lower circulating levels of angiotensin-converting enzyme (ACE) in patients with schizophrenia', *Schizophrenia Research*, 2018.

Mrug et al., 'Sodium and potassium excretion predict increased depression in urban adolescents', *Physiological Reports*, 2019.

Musch et al., 'Solute loss plays a major role in polydipsia-related hyponatraemia of both water drinkers and beer drinkers', *Quarterly Journal of Medicine*, 2003.

Natelson et al., 'Physiological assessment of orthostatic intolerance in chronic fatigue syndrome', *Journal of Translational Medicine*, 2022.

Naviaux et al., 'Metabolic features of chronic fatigue syndrome', *Proceedings of the National Academy of Sciences of the United States of America*, 2016.

Noakes T., *Waterlogged: The Serious Problem of Overhydration in Endurance Sports*, Human Kinetics, 2012.

Nunes et al., 'Ionic imbalance, in addition to molecular crowding, abates cytoskeletal dynamics and vesicle motility during hypertonic stress', *Proceedings of the National Academy of Sciences of the United States of America*, 2015.

Pretorius et al., 'The Occurrence of Hyperactivated Platelets and Fibrinaloid Microclots in Myalgic Encephalomyelitis/Chronic Fatigue Syndrome (ME/CFS)', *Pharmaceuticals (Basel)*, 2022.

Ramirez and Graham, 'Hiccups, Compulsive Water Drinking, and Hyponatremia', *Annals of Internal Medicine*, 1993.

Raj et al., 'Renin-Aldosterone paradox and perturbed blood volume regulation underlying postural tachycardia syndrome', *Circulation*, 2005.

Robbins and Carter, 'The Use of Hypertonic Saline Infusions in the Differential Diagnosis of Diabetes Insipidus and Psychogenic Polydipsia', *Journal of Clinical Endocrinology and Metabolism*, 1947.

Robertson, 'Dipsogenic diabetes insipidus: a newly recognized syndrome caused by a selective defect in the osmoregulation of thirst', *Transactions of the Association of American Physicians*, 1987.

Robinson et al., 'The Influence of Dietary Salt Beyond Blood Pressure', *Current Hypertension Reports*, 2019.

Rowe, 'General Information Brochure on Orthostatic Intolerance and its Treatment' (website: https://www.dysautonomiainternational.org/pdf/RoweOIsummary.pdf).

Rubin et al., 'Reduced Levels of Vasopressin and Reduced Behavioural Modulation of Oxytocin in Psychotic Disorders', *Schizophrenia Bulletin*, 2014.

Ruzieh et al., 'Effects of intermittent intravenous saline infusions in patients with medication-refractory postural tachycardia syndrome', *Journal of Interventional Cardiac Electrophysiology*, 2017.

Sailer et al., 'Primary Polydipsia in the medical and psychiatric patient: characteristics, complications and therapy', *Swiss Medical Weekly*, 2017.

Sarai and Matsunaga 'ADH secretion in schizophrenic patients on antipsychotic drugs', *Biological Psychiatry*, 1989.

Saruta et al., 'Evaluation of the renin-angiotensin system in diabetes insipidus and psychogenic polydipsia', *Nephron*, 1982.

Schaterlee et al., 'A comparison of pregnancies that occur before and after the onset of chronic fatigue syndrome', *Archives of Internal Medicine*, 2004.

Scheibenbogen and Wirth, 'Pathophysiology of skeletal muscle disturbances in Myalgic Encephalomyelitis/Chronic Fatigue Syndrome (ME/CFS)', *Journal of Translational Medicine*, 2021.

Scheibenbogen, Wirth and Paul, 'An attempt to explain the neurological symptoms of Myalgic Encephalomyelitis/Chronic Fatigue Syndrome', *Journal of Translational Medicine*, 2021.

Scheibenbogen and Wirth, 'A Unifying Hypothesis of the Pathophysiology of Myalgic Encephalomyelitis/Chronic Fatigue Syndrome (ME/CFS): Recognitions from the finding of autoantibodies against ß2-adrenergic receptors', *Autoimmunity Reviews*, 2020.

Selvarajah, 'Skin Sodium and Hypertension: A Paradigm Shift?', *Current Hypertension Reports*, 2019.

Scott et al., 'Small adrenal glands in chronic fatigue syndrome: a preliminary computer tomography study', *Psychoneuroendocrinology*, 1999.

Shan et al., 'Neuroimaging characteristics of myalgic encephalomyelitis/chronic fatigue syndrome (ME/CFS): a systematic review', *Journal of Translational Medicine*, 2020.

Shan et al., 'Multimodal MRI of myalgic encephalomyelitis/chronic fatigue syndrome: a cross-sectional neuroimaging study toward its neuropathophysiology and diagnosis', *Frontiers in Neurology*, 2022.

Streeten and Bell, 'The roles of orthostatic hypotension, orthostatic tachycardia, and subnormal erythrocyte volume in the pathogenesis of the chronic fatigue syndrome', *The American Journal of the Medical Sciences*, 2000.

Subramanian et al., 'Converging Neurobiological Evidence in Primary Polydipsia Resembling Obsessive Compulsive Disorder', *Indian Journal of Psychological Medicine*, 2017.

Thaweethai et al., 'Development of a Definition of Post-acute Sequelae of SARS-CoV-2 Infection', *JAMA*, 2023.

Titze et al., 'Increased salt consumption induces body water conservation and decreases fluid intake', *Journal of Clinical Investigation*, 2017.

Tomas et al., 'A Review of Hypothalamic-Pituitary-Adrenal Axis Function in Chronic Fatigue Syndrome', *ISRN Neuroscience*, 2013.

Torres-Harding et al., 'The associations between basal salivary cortisol and illness symptomatology in chronic fatigue syndrome', *Journal of applied biobehavioral research*, 2008.

Utzon et al., 'Psychogenic polydipsia: pronounced cerebral edema after exaggerated consumption of boiled water', *Ugeskr Laeger*, 1991.

Walker M., *Skewed: Psychiatric Hegemony and the Manufacture of Mental Illness in Multiple Chemical Sensitivity, Gulf War Syndrome, Myalgic Encephalomyelitis and Chronic Fatigue Syndrome*, Sling-Shot Press, 2003.

Wedeen R., 'Prolonged Functional Depression of Antidiuretic Hormone, *Journal of Psychiatry & Neuroscience*, 1961.

Weir and Speight, 'ME/CFS: Past, Present and Future', *Healthcare*, 2021.

Wenstedt et al., 'Effect of high-salt diet on blood pressure and body fluid composition in patients with type 1 diabetes: randomized controlled intervention trial', *BMJ Open Diabetes Research & Care*, 2020.

Venkatesan et al., 'A Subset of Primary Polydipsia, "Dipsogenic Diabetes Insipidus", in Apparently Healthy People Due to Excessive Water Intake: Not Enough Light to Illuminate the Dark Tunnel', *Healthcare*, 2021.

Vermino et al., 'Postural orthostatic tachycardia syndrome (POTS): State of the science and clinical care from a 2019 National Institutes of Health Expert Consensus Meeting – Part 1', *Autonomic Neuroscience*, 2021.

Vieweg, 'Psychogenic polydipsia and water intoxication--concepts that have failed', *Biological Psychiatry*, 1985.

Visser and Van Campen, 'Blood Volume Status in Patients with Chronic Fatigue Syndrome: Relation to Complaints', *Frontiers in Pediatrics*, 2018.

Visser and Van Campen, 'Deconditioning does not explain orthostatic intolerance in ME/CFS (myalgic encephalomyelitis/chronic fatigue syndrome')', *Journal of Translational Medicine*, 2021.

Visser and Van Campen, 'Orthostatic Intolerance in Long-Haul COVID after SARS-CoV-2: A Case-Control Comparison with Post-EBV and Insidious-Onset Myalgic Encephalomyelitis/Chronic Fatigue Syndrome Patients', *Healthcare*, 2022.

Yasuoka et al., 'Effects of Angiotensin II on Erythropoietin Production in the Kidney and Liver', *Molecules*, 2021.

Printed in Great Britain
by Amazon

37297303R00096